Hair Cell Micromechanics
and
Otoacoustic Emissions

Hair Cell Micromechanics
and
Otoacoustic Emissions

Edited by

Charles I. Berlin, PhD
Linda J. Hood, PhD
Anthony Ricci, PhD

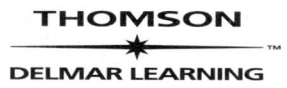

THOMSON

DELMAR LEARNING

Australia Canada Mexico Singapore Spain United Kingdom United States

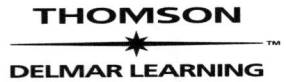

Hair Cell Micromechanics and Otoacoustic Emissions
Edited by Charles I. Berlin, PhD, Linda J. Hood, PhD, and Anthony Ricci, PhD

Business Unit Director:
William Brottmiller

Developmental Editor:
Juliet Byington

Production Editor:
James Zayicek

Executive Editor:
Cathy L. Esperti

Editorial Assistant:
Maria D'Angelico

Project Editor:
Bryan Viggiani

Acquisitions Editor:
Candice Janco

Executive Marketing Manager:
Dawn F. Gerrain

Production Coordinator:
Nina Lontrato

For permission to use material from this text or product, contact us by
Tel (800) 730-2214
Fax (800) 730-2215
www.thomsonrights.com

Library of Congress Cataloging-in-Publication Data
Hair cell micromechanics and otoacoustic emissions / edited by Charles I. Berlin, Linda J. Hood, Anthony Ricci.
    p. cm.
Includes bibliographical references and index.
    ISBN: 0-7668-6190-2 (alk. paper)
    1. Hair cells. 2. Otoacoustic emissions. I. Berlin, Charles I. II. Hood, Linda J. III. Ricci, Anthony.
    QP471.2 .H37 2002
    573.8'919--dc21

2002019370

Contents

Preface

This is the seventh book in the Kresge-Mirmelstein Award cycle published and supported by Thomson-Delmar Learning. The series was conceived by the late Rona Mirmelstein, a great benefactor of the Kresge Lab, and Dr. Charles Berlin. Mrs. Mirmelstein's daughter, Karyl Ann "Kam" Mirmelstein Lemberger, has also created a professorship at Kresge in her mother's name. Each year, The Kresge Lab gives a cash prize to a peer-selected scientist who has made a singularly powerful and original contribution to hearing science. At the awarding of the prize, a full day of talks are presented, orchestrated around the prize winner's topic. The talks become chapters, and the chapters become books like these. This is the seventh in the series and celebrates Peter Dallos for his isolation and cloning of Prestin, the motor that drives the outer hair cell. Dallos' award was presented on October 27, 2000. He was selected to receive the prize by a truly august panel—the previous six winners, each listed below.

1. William Brownell won initially for his discovery of outer hair cell motility; his seminar led to the now-classic book *Hair Cells and Hearing Aids*, published in 1996. The volume contained an audio CD sponsored by Mead Killion and Etymotic Research, which demonstrated many of the principles outlined in the chapters and also contained examples of degraded speech meant to simulate hearing loss.
2. The next prize in the series was awarded to Robert Wenthold for his studies in the biochemistry of the ear. His presentation led to a book entitled *Neurotransmission and Hearing Loss*, published in 1996.
3. The third winner was David Kemp, the discoverer of otoacoustic emissions. His presentation led to a book called *Otoacoustic Emissions* and celebrated the 25th anniversary of his discovery. The book was among the first in our field to have an interactive CD with a working model of the basilar membrane, which allowed the user to extract distortion products from a nonlinear cochlear partition and demonstrate the shift of cochlear partition location with frequency.

4. The fourth winner was M. Charles Liberman whose presentation led to a book called *The Efferent System* with a video CD created by Jont Allen of Bell Telephone Labs. Allen summarized a unique theory of cochlear tuning with a model made of rubber bands and counterweights that demonstrated how both high and low pass filtering could operate in the same location of the cochlear partition based on relative changes of stiffness of the various portions of the organ of Corti, outer hair cells, and tectorial membrane, which control their respective shearing forces.

5. Karen Steel, of the MRC Hearing Research Institute, won the next prize for her contribution to the understanding of the genetics of hearing loss. The volume was co-edited by Dr. Bronya Keats and featured a CD that described a Balinese culture whose members all used an indigenous sign language because many of the inhabitants were deaf. Since all the villagers used the language, deafness was not a serious social handicap. The CD also had examples of how people in our culture adapt to deafness, using sign language, cued speech, or combinations thereof. The examples, both Balinese and Western, were presented for the benefit of hearing scientists who would otherwise not be exposed to the social and cultural impact of the deafness they studied in the laboratory. The Balinese videos were supplied by Drs. Tom Friedman and John T. Hinnant.

6. David Corey of Harvard was selected by his peers for the sixth prize because of his landmark work in studying hair cell motility, their channels and methods of adaptation, and because he had participated in studies linking a myosin gene in the Shaker-1 mouse to one form of Usher syndrome. The volume, co-edited by Dr. Richard P. Bobbin, featured studies of mammalian hair cells as well as a living hair cell organism, the sea anemone, whose function required intact calcium channels in much the same way as mammalian hair cells.

ABOUT THIS VOLUME

This volume features and honors the work of Dr. Peter Dallos. He was selected by the previous Kresge-Mirmelstein award winners for his cloning of Prestin, a gene that contributes to cellular motility. His paper was complemented by outstanding summaries of hair cell adaptation and molecular chemistry by Drs. Bobbin and Ricci, genetics of Usher syndrome by Dr. Keats, the modulation of the resting potassium current in type I vestibular hair cells by Dr. Rennie, clinical applications of otoacoustic emissions by Dr. Hood, and the physiological bases of audiological management by Dr. Berlin. What gives this book its unique time-binding quality is that Dr. William Brownell, the first winner, returned to show how cellular motility is traceable phylogenetically to prehistoric motile bacteria. These primitive simple organisms used ball bearing-like molecular properties to move, and may have set the stage for contractile lattices specific to the cochlea. For the clinical readers, we also presented data on the audiologic manifestations of genetic hearing loss and information on using the physiology of the cochlea to better understand the various diagnostic options that face us.

The CD included with this book reviews and highlights the physiologic properties of the mammalian cochlea that can be measured both in humans and other animals. The demonstrations formulate the basis of Dr. Berlin's chapter on the physiological bases of audiological evaluation. The CD demonstrates cochlear microphonics, action potentials, and summating potentials as well as otoacoustic emissions for readers who might have only limited familiarity with them.

It was all in all a thrilling scientific day that led to this volume and set the stage for future compilations.

Each year we continue to thank Dr. Berlin's benefactress, Frances Barnes Bullington, for her unflagging generosity and support of our work, and her legacy of funding both a Professorship and a Chair as described in the following. She has been a steadfast and faithful supporter of our laboratory and will be instrumental in assuring its survival. Our deepest gratitude to you.

The editors,

Charles I. Berlin, PhD
Kenneth and Frances Barnes Bullington Professor of Hearing Science
Professor Otolaryngology Head and Neck Surgery
Director Kresge Hearing Research Laboratory of the South
cberli@lsuhsc.edu

Linda J. Hood, PhD, Professor

Anthony Ricci, PhD, Assistant Professor

Acknowledgments

These volumes and prizes were conceived by Dr. Charles Berlin and Rona Becker Mirmelstein to celebrate the restoration of the hearing abilities of her daughter Karyl Ann "Kam" Mirmelstein Lemberger. The volumes honor and reward scientists studying auditory mechanisms and whose work leads to germinal changes in our understanding of hearing. We thank Kam who has also started a Professorship in her mother's name to perpetuate this prize. We also thank our many other supporters throughout the years, including NIH, DRF, NOHR, NSF, the Marriott, Oberkotter and Lions Eye Foundations, as well as the Foundation of the LSU Health Sciences Center.

The support of our Department Head, Dr. Daniel Nuss, and the administration of LSU HSC facilitates advances like this; we especially appreciate, but will miss, the support of our late Chancellor Mervin L. Trail, MD, who died suddenly in January 2001. He will be sorely missed.

The editing and organization skills of Bobby Moore and Susan Stauss have helped complete this volume in a timely fashion, and we are especially indebted to them. We are also grateful to our authors and the Thomson-Delmar Learning staff.

List of Contributors

Charles I. Berlin, PhD
Kresge Hearing Research
    Laboratory
Department of Otorhinolaryngology
Louisiana State University Health
    Sciences Center
New Orleans, Louisiana

Richard P. Bobbin, PhD
Kresge Hearing Research
    Laboratory of the South
Department of Otorhinolaryngology
    and Biocommunication
Louisiana State University Health
    Sciences Center
New Orleans, Louisiana

Shanda Brashears, MCD
Kresge Hearing Research
    Laboratory of the South
Department of Otorhinolaryngology
    and Biocommunication
Louisiana State University Health
    Sciences Center
New Orleans, Louisiana

W. E. Brownell, PhD
Bobby R. Alford Department of
    Otorhinolaryngology and
    Communicative Sciences
Baylor College of Medicine
Houston, Texas

Julie Campbell, BS
Kresge Hearing Research
    Laboratory of the South
Department of Otorhinolaryngology
    and Biocommunication
Louisiana State University Health
    Sciences Center
New Orleans, Louisiana

Peter Dallos, PhD
Northwestern University
Auditory Physiology Laboratory
    (the Hugh Knowles Center)
Departments of Neurobiology and
    Physiology and Communication
    Sciences and Disorders
The Institute of Neuroscience
Evanston, Illinois

Linda J. Hood, PhD
Kresge Hearing Research
    Laboratory
Department of Otorhinolaryngology
Louisiana State University Health
    Sciences Center
New Orleans, Louisiana

Jennifer Jeanfreau, MCD
Kresge Hearing Research
    Laboratory of the South
Department of Otorhinolaryngology
    and Biocommunication
Louisiana State University Health
    Sciences Center
New Orleans, Louisiana

Bronya J. B. Keats, PhD
Department of Genetics
Louisiana State University
    Health Sciences Center
New Orleans, Louisiana

Suzanne Lousteau
Kresge Hearing Research
    Laboratory of the South
Department of Otorhinolaryngology
    and Biocommunication
Louisiana State University Health
    Sciences Center
New Orleans, Louisiana

Manisha Mandhare, BS
Kresge Hearing Research
    Laboratory of the South
Department of Otorhinolaryngology
    and Biocommunication
Louisiana State University Health
    Sciences Center
New Orleans, Louisiana

Thierry Morlet, PhD
Kresge Hearing Research
    Laboratory of the South
Department of Otorhinolaryngology
    and Biocommunication
Louisiana State University Health
    Sciences Center
New Orleans, Louisiana

K. J. Rennie, PhD
Department of Otolaryngology
University of Texas Medical Branch
Galveston, Texas

Anthony Ricci, PhD
Neuroscience Center of Excellence
    and Kresge Hearing Lab
Louisiana State University Health
    Sciences Center
New Orleans, Louisiana

Sevtap Savas, PhD
Department of Genetics
Louisiana State University Health
    Sciences Center
New Orleans, Louisiana

Outer Hair Cell: The Key to Mammalian Hearing

Peter Dallos, PhD
Northwestern University
Auditory Physiology Laboratory (the Hugh Knowles Center)
Departments of Neurobiology and Physiology
and Communication Sciences and Disorders,
The Institute for Neuroscience
Evanston, Illinois

INTRODUCTION

Sensory receptor cells of the ear were first seen by Corti (1851), and their stereociliary bundle was first observed by Hensen (1863). It was also Hensen who suggested that the stereocilia play an important role in the excitation of these cells. While it was recognized that two morphologically different receptors of hair cell types coexisted in the mammalian cochlea, similar function was assigned to them. Only in the 1950s and 1960s, when ultrastructural studies (Engström, 1958; Engström Ades, & Hawkins, 1962; Kimura, 1966) began revealing significant differences between the two sensory cell types, and, more importantly, when their innervation patterns were shown to be radically different (Smith & Sjöstrand, 1961a, 1961b; Spoendlin, 1966, 1969), did the first ideas emerge that inner and outer hair cells may have different functions. Even then, if there were a viewpoint at all, it was that, in some loose analogy to the dichotomy of retinal photoreceptors, outer hair cells (OHC) somehow served low-level hearing and inner hair cells (IHC) processed high-level sounds. In excellent handbook chapters and authoritative reviews at the mid-20th century mark, one is hard-pressed to find discussions that treat the two types of hair cells as distinct functional entities. What might now be considered as one of auditory periphery's focal points, the role and operation of the two kinds of hair cells, is an enterprise less than 50 years old.

Arguably, it was Hallowell Davis who, in the late 1950s, introduced the notion that the two hair cell types respond to different mechanical stimulation (Davis, 1959, 1960). He related the finding that cochlear microphonic (CM) potentials could better be associated with outer hair cells while summating potentials (SP) with inner hair cells (Davis et al., 1958) to some of Békésy's observations on the local direction of movements of the tectorial membrane. Davis proposed that, "we should think of the cochlea as composed of two sensory systems side by side. The external hair cells are a sensitive, fragile system while the internal hair cells are a less sensitive but much more rugged system" (Davis, 1960, pp. 35–36). In other words, while Davis based his contentions on experimental evidence currently available, in his thinking the division of the sound-intensity range between the two cell types remained their principal raison d'être. Davis' early work, in which he used ototoxic antibiotics to produce documented hair cell damage in order to assess IHC and OHC function, was followed by similar efforts in the 1960s and 1970s by a number of groups. There were two notable early contributions that set the tone for subsequent work. Kiang, Maxon, and Levine (1970) pioneered recording single auditory nerve fiber discharges in connection with inducing hair cell damage with streptomyces antibiotics. While this work could say little about differential influences by the two hair cell populations on account of the experimental animals' (cats) tendency to lose both their OHCs and IHCs together, the work presaged experiments that laid the foundation of current thinking. The other experimental work pertained to functional differences between the two hair cell types. This work was founded on theoretical suggestions that IHCs should respond to basilar membrane velocity (Billone & Raynor, 1973) based on anatomical observations of a lack of firm contact between their stereocilia and the tectorial membrane (Engström et al., 1962; Lim, 1972; Lindemann, Ades, Bredberg, & Engström, 1971). It was indeed found when measuring cochlear potentials in guinea pigs after kanamycin administration, that the residual CM response, presumably produced by IHCs, reflected the time derivative of basilar-membrane displacement (Dallos, 1973; Dallos, Billone, Durrant, Wang, & Raynor, 1972).

In the 1970s, a flurry of activity followed these early efforts, and two main avenues were taken. In the first, the work of Davis and colleagues (Davis et al., 1958) on apportioning the sources of CM and SP was followed up (Dallos & Cheatham, 1976; Dallos & Wang, 1974). The second initiated the quest for experimentally determining the role of OHCs in hearing. With the advent of understanding the highly assymmetrical afferent innervation of OHCs and IHCs (Spoendlin, 1969), old notions of low- versus high-level sound processing by the two hair cell populations had quietly expired. Inner hair cells clearly conveyed essentially all, if not all, sound-related information to the brain. At the same time, the concept of cochlear amplification became established, and OHCs became implicated in this process. The research of this period has been reviewed (Dallos, 1985, 1988), and a detailed examination is not warranted. However, certain key ideas, relevant to the present concerns and their experimental foundations, are worth restating.

During the early 1970s, several lines of thought dominated auditory research. One of the most powerful, but unfortunately based on inadequate experimental data, was the perceived need of filtering/ amplification between basilar membrane motion and auditory nerve fiber responses (Evans & Wilson, 1973). Even though clear indications were unavailable that basilar membrane response was nonlinear (Rhode, 1971) and physiologically vulnerable (Khollöffel, 1972; Rhode, 1973), the idea persisted that its characteristics could not account for the properties of neural responses. Because of this, a variety of schemes, many of them invoking neural interactions between fibers coming from IHCs and OHCs, were proposed (Evans & Wilson, 1973; Lynn & Sayers, 1970; Zwislocki, 1974, 1977) in the spirit of Békésy's (1960) notion of neural funneling. We note that while these ideas were based on false premises, they nevertheless represent the first suggestion that there needs to be an interaction between the OHC and IHC systems in order to produce normal cochlear response. Based on experiments using OHC destruction by the administration of kanamycin, Ryan and Dallos (1975) and Dallos and Harris (1978) first proposed direct interactions between OHCs and IHCs: "the OHCs are specialized to perform a facilitatory function on the IHCs" (Ryan & Dallos, 1975, p. 45), and "outer hair cells provide a frequency-dependent sensitizing influence to the inner hair cells" (Dallos & Harris, 1978, p. 365). Furthermore, it was suggested that the origin of prominent nonlinear processes that characterize cochlear operation are found in OHCs: "nonlinear phenomena originate in an interplay of electrical and mechanical processes in the hair cells whose cilia maintain intimate contact with the tectorial membrane. It appears to us that in the mammalian cochlea these cells are the outer hair cells" (Dallos, Harris, Relkin, & Cheatham, 1980, p. 247). Thus, two-tone supression and distortion product (e.g., 2f1-f2) production are correlated with the integrity of OHCs (Dallos et al., 1980; Schmiedt, Zwislocki, & Hamernik, 1980). The fact that prominent nonlinear distortion in the cochlea was associated with hair cell sources was surmised from early psychophysical experiments by Goldstein (1967) and from electrophysiological experiments by Dallos, Schoeny, Worthington, and Cheatham (1969). Examples from some key experiments are shown in Figures 1–1 to 1–4 for reference.

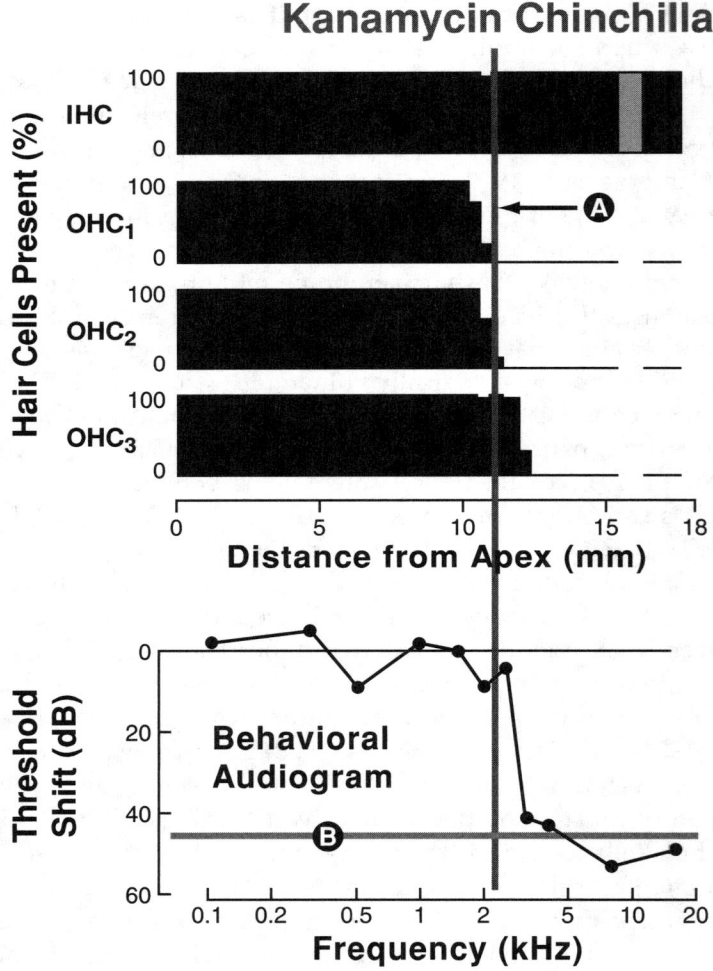

Figure 1–1. Top: cytocochleogram showing percent of hair cells present as a function of cochlear location. Bottom: behavioral audiogram showing threshold shift corresponding to OHC loss. **A**-line: approximate boundary of OHC lesion. **B**-line: approximate threshold shift corresponding to the lesion. Modified from Ryan and Dallos, 1975.

Kanamycin Chinchilla

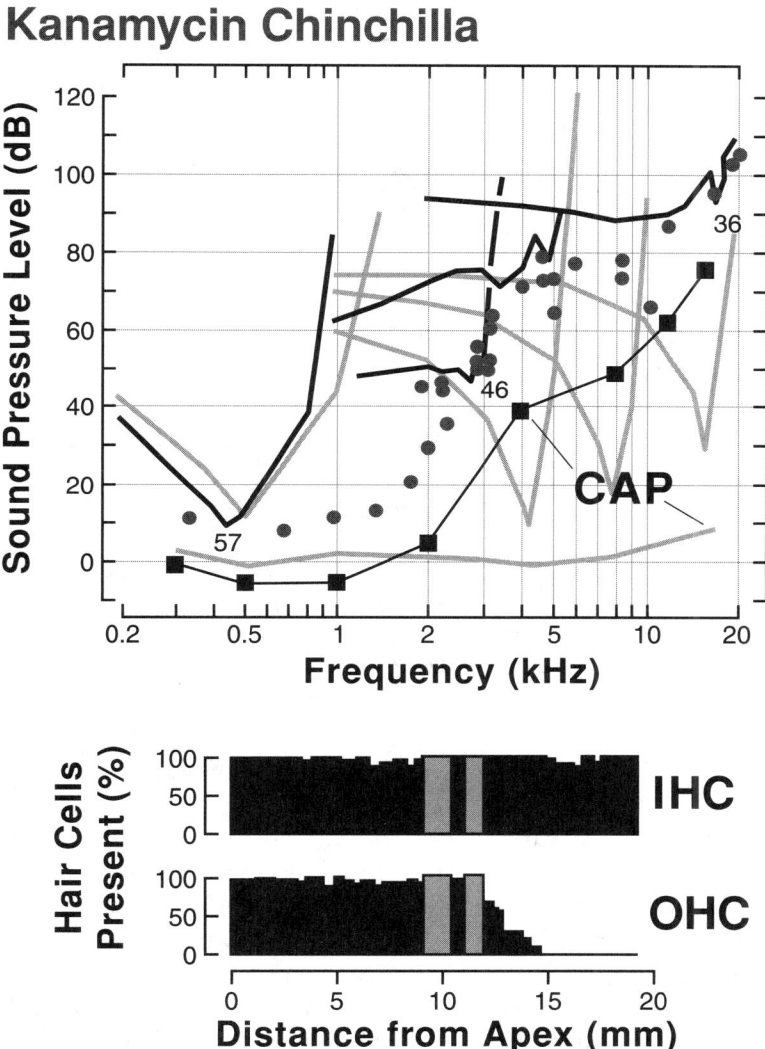

Figure 1–2. Bottom: cytocochleogram. Top: auditory nerve responses. CAP: compound action potential thresholds for this animal (thin black line with square data points) and average normal (gray line). Round dots: individual fiber thresholds at best frequency. Black lines: example of complete tuning curves for this animal, in comparison to representative normal tuning curves having the same best frequency (gray line). Modified from Dallos and Harris, 1978.

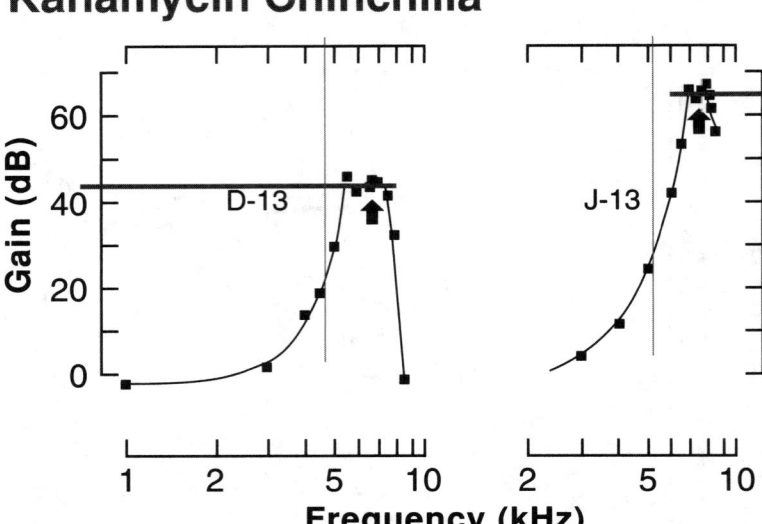

Figure 1–3. Two examples of the decibel difference between single unit tuning curves obtained from OHC-deprived cochleas (as in Figure 1–2) and normal tuning curves of the same characteristic frequency. The difference is interpreted as the gain supplied by OHCs. Modified from Dallos and Harris, 1978.

DISCOVERY OF MECHANICAL FEEDBACK

The mechanical nature of the previously mentioned interaction emerged from various lines of experimentation. Included are the discovery of otoacoustic emissions (Kemp, 1978), effects of stimulation of the efferent system (Brown & Nuttal, 1984; Mountain, 1980; Siegel & Kim, 1982), and, owing to improved techniques, the gradual disappearance of discrepancies between basilar membrane and neural tuning (Khanna & Leonard, 1982; Robels, Ruggero, & Rich, 1986; Sellick, Patuzzi, & Johnstone, 1982). In fact, contemporary recordings indicate that in the best frequency region there is a quantitative agreement between basilar membrane and neural responses (Narayan, Temchin, Recio, & Ruggero, 1998).

What cemented the notion of mechanical feedback from OHCs to basilar membrane, representing a process of amplification, was the discovery of OHC electromotility by Brownell (Brownell, 1983; Brownell, Bader, Bertrand, & deRibaupierre, 1985; Kachar, Brownell,

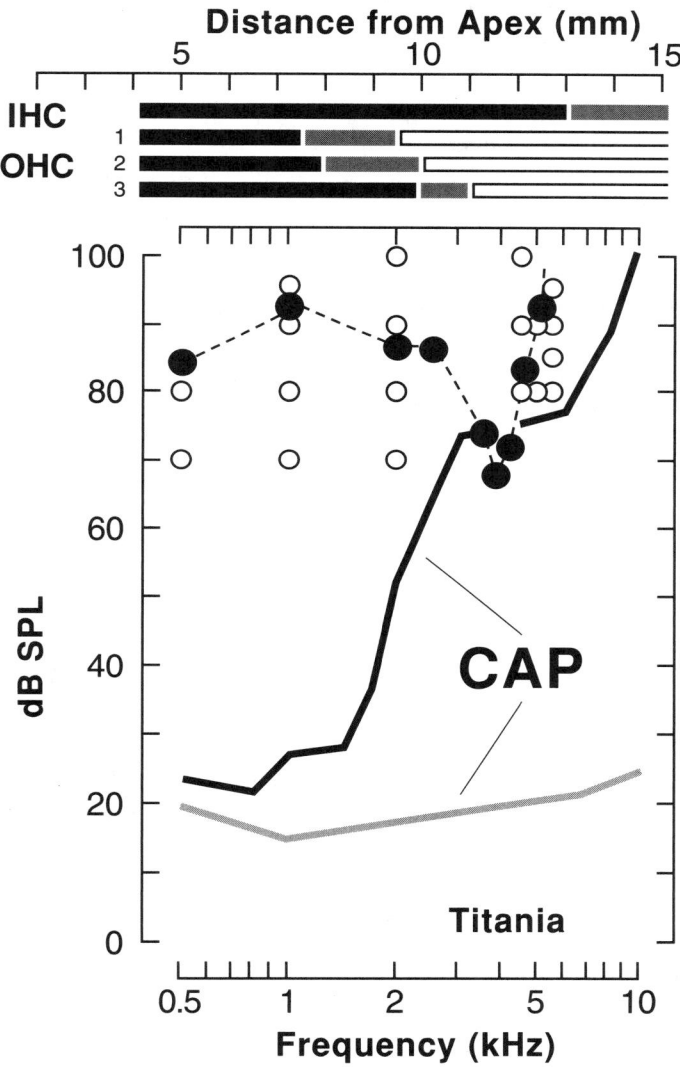

Figure 1–4. Top: cytocochleogram. Bottom: Compound action potential thresholds. Thick black line: this animal. Thick gray line: average normal. Dotted line with dots: single fiber threshold. Open circles: sound frequency/level combinations that did *not* produce two-tone suppression. Modified from Dallos et al., 1980.

Altschuler, & Fex, 1986). This feedback process became widely accepted and modeled during the 15 years subsequent to its discovery (reviews: Dallos, 1992; Holley, 1996; Patuzzi, 1996). While electromotile feedback from OHCs is an appealing idea, certain difficulties with its operation have been pointed out over time. One of these pertains to the efficiency of coupling axial OHC contraction-expansion cycles to the radial displacement of the reticular lamina (Hudspeth, 1989, 1997). The other problem is that inasmuch as electromotility is membrane-voltage dependent (Santos-Sacchi & Dilger, 1988) and the OHC membrane constitutes a low-pass filter (Santos-Sacchi, 1992), there is doubt that there remains a sufficiently large receptor potential at high frequencies to drive effectively the electromotile process. These difficulties remain, in spite of considerable success in modeling the feedback process (Kolston, 1999) and suggestions of how the system might overcome the "low-pass filter problem" (Dallos & Evans, 1995; Mountain & Hubbard, 1994).

AMPLIFICATION PROCESS

One aspect of the cochlea's operation that is frequently evoked as proof of the existence of an amplification process is spontaneous otoacoustic emissions (Kemp, 1979; Wilson, 1980). However, inasmuch as such emissions can be recorded from the ears of essentially all vertebrates, not only mammals, it is said that amplification cannot generally be tied to OHCs that are a mammalian specialization (for review, see Manley & Köppl, 1998). Instead, mechanisms related to mechanoelectrical transducer (MET) function are now considered by many to be the common substrate of amplification in ears (Choe, Magnasco, & Hudspeth, 1998; Martin & Hudspeth, 1999; Ricci, Crawford, & Fettiplace, 2000). In spite of all the work on OHC motility, it is still unproven that the dominant effector in the amplification process is in fact somatic motility, even in mammals. Another possibility is some form of ciliary motility or impedance change (Benser et al., 1996; Hudspeth, 1989; Martin & Hudspeth, 1999; Mountain, Hubbard, & McMullen, 1983). There are examples of ciliary motility in nonmammalian hair cells (Assad, Hacohen, & Corey, 1989; Benser et al., 1996; Crawford & Fettiplace, 1985; Martin & Hudspeth, 1999), as well as theoretical constructs showing that such motility can provide amplification (Camalet, Duke, Julicher, & Prost, 2000; Eguiluz, Ospeck, Choe, Hudspeth, & Magnasco, 2000; Martin & Hudspeth, 1999). Virtually all vertebrates are capable of producing otoacoustic emissions (Köppl, 1995; Probst, 1990; Probst, Lansbury-Martin, & Martin, 1991; Van Dijk, Manly, & Gallo, 1998). Because it has been assumed that emissions are a signature of the amplifier's operation, their presence in animals lacking OHCs (hence somatic motility) is construed as an argument for ciliary amplification. As early as 1986, Kim proposed a dual mechanism in which both somatic and ciliary motility contribute to the amplification process.

It appears likely that an amplifier based on MET processes eliminates the difficulty with providing adequate gain at high frequencies. However, it is unclear how concomitant stereocilia bundle motions would couple back to exert significant influence on basilar membrane displacement. This is an essential requirement due to the virtual identity of basilar membrane and neural tuning curves in the mammal (Narayan et al., 1998).

To appreciate the need for amplification, consider vibratory amplitudes at threshold. Extrapolations of eardrum displacement to the approximate threshold of 0 dB SPL yields approximately 1 pm (Guinan & Peake, 1967). From basilar membrane motions at the same sound level (Ruggero, Rich, Recio, Narayan, & Robles, 1997; Sellick et al., 1982) and with the assumption of no significant mechanical gain between basilar membrane and ciliary displacement, one obtains ~0.3 nm for the latter. There is a need for some 50 dB mechanical gain in displacement amplitude as shown in Figure 1–5. Even after such amplification, ciliary displacement is extremely small (equivalent to displacing the top of the Sears Tower by 2 inches). However, to achieve similar cilia motion without amplification, one would have to increase sound level input to the ear by some 50 dB.

While it remains unproven that OHC motility constitutes the basis of cochlear amplification, the phenomenon itself is sufficiently interesting and unique in biology to merit continued consideration, and it is the subject of the remainder of this chapter.

OUTER HAIR CELL MOTILITY

Studies of the OHC electromotile response have established some of its fundamental behaviors (Ashmore, 1987; Kachar et al., 1986). It depends on membrane potential, as opposed to membrane current (Iwasa & Kachar, 1989; Santos-Sacchi & Dilger, 1988). It is also independent of aerobic and anaerobic metabolism (Brownell et al., 1985;

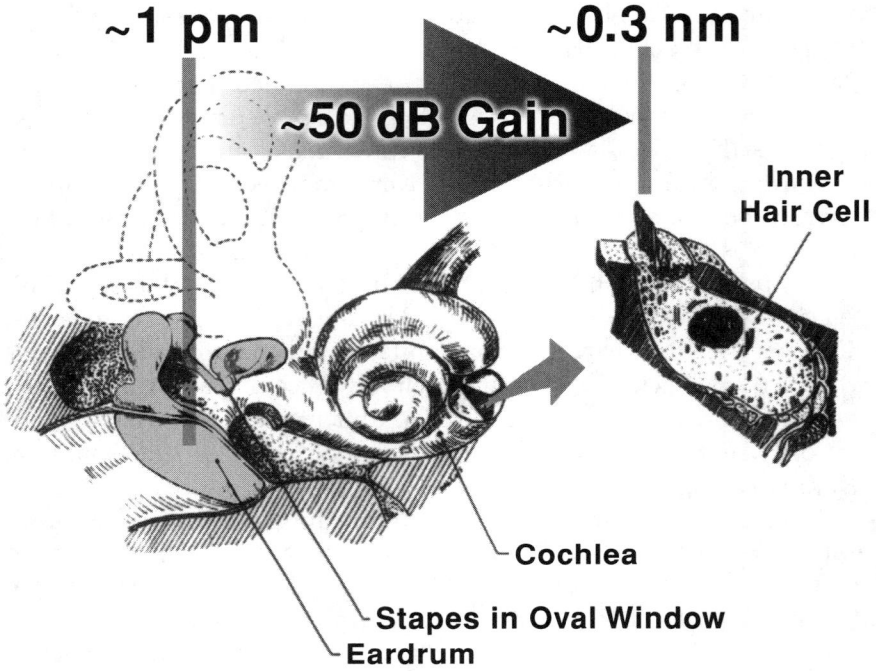

Figure 1–5. Illustration demonstrating amplification of vibrations from the eardrum to the stereocilia of IHCs. The indicated amplitudes are at the threshold of hearing at frequencies where the ear is most sensitive.

Holley & Ashmore, 1988a; Kachar et al., 1986) and of calcium (Ashmore, 1987; Santos-Sacchi, 1989). OHC motility is nonlinear because its displacement response to a sinusoidal voltage command contains a direct current (DC) component (Evans, Dallos, & Hallworth, 1989, 1991; Santos-Sacchi, 1989), plus harmonic (Santos-Sacchi, 1992) and intermodulation (Hu, Evans, He, & Dallos, 1994) distortion. Electromotile responses are also associated with charge displacement currents that manifest themselves as voltage-dependent nonlinear capacitance (NLC; Ashmore, 1989; Santos-Sacchi, 1991). NLC is now commonly used as the signature of OHC motility. Other studies suggest that both the motor and its sensor are located in the plasma membrane, as opposed to the elaborate cortical lattice structure (Huang & Santos-Sacchi, 1993; Kalinec, Holley, Iwasa, Lim, & Kachar, 1992). The most likely candidates for the elementary motors are the large, ~10 nm diameter, protein particles with packing densities exceeding 5,000 μm^{-2}, that cover as much as 75% of the plasma membrane (Forge, 1991; Kalinec et al., 1992). It is possible that the large particles are multimers of the minor protein prestin (see below).

MOTILITY'S DISTINGUISHING FEATURE

Probably the most distinguishing feature of motility is that the rate of change of cell shape is very high. Early measurements demonstrated that the rate constant of the process was in the millisecond range (Santos-Sacchi, 1992). Dallos and Evans (1995) showed that if the electrical low-pass filter properties of the cell membrane were neutralized, electromotility could be measured without diminution up to ~24 kHz (the limit imposed by their equipment). These results implied that the rate constant of the motile process itself is less than 10 μsec and probably considerably less. Subsequently, Gale and Ashmore (1997) made the contrary suggestion that the motility possesses a distinct "speed limit" of about 25 kHz. This was shown not to be the case by Frank, Hemmet, and Gummer (1999) who measured motility above 70 kHz. It is probably true that the motile process itself is capable of operating at any frequency where mammalian hearing is functional.

Electromotility In Situ

Other measurements of electromotility in situ prove that OHCs are capable of displacing the basilar membrane-organ of Corti complex (Mammano & Ashmore, 1993; Nuttal & Dolan, 1993; Xue et al., 1993). Somatic motility occurs upon deflection of the stereociliary bundle (Evans & Dallos, 1993), suggesting that the OHC can affect micromechanics via its own receptor potential. This possibility made it important to determine and manipulate the static axial stiffness of OHCs (Gitter, Rudert, & Zenner, 1993; Hallworth, 1995; He & Dallos, 2000; Holley & Ashmore, 1988b; Iwasa & Adachi, 1997; Russel & Schauz, 1995; Tolomeo, Steele, & Holley, 1996; Ulfendahl et al., 1998). Experimental evidence indicates that axial stiffness and electromotility are correlated; both depend on membrane potential and both are reduced by gadolinium (He & Dallos, 1999, 2000). It is also known that axial stiffness receives contributions from both the plasma membrane and cortical lattice (Oghalai, Patel, Nakagawa, & Brownell, 1998; Tolomeo et al., 1996).

Electromotility In Vivo

A modulatory influence on OHC electromotility in vivo is probably provided by the OHCs' efferent innervation because medial olivo-cochlear efferents end almost exclusively on OHCs (Eybalin, 1993; Guinan, 1996). Electrical stimulation of efferent fibers or perfusion of the scala tympani with acetylcholine (ACh) reduces sound-evoked responses at best frequency (Galambos, 1956; Murugasu & Russell, 1996; Sridhar, Liberman, Brown, & Sewell, 1995). Evidence suggests that ACh binds to a special nicotinic ACh receptor (nAChR) that shows mixed nicotinic and muscarinic pharmacological properties (Guth & Norris, 1996, for review). This receptor subtype, the $\alpha 9$, when expressed in oocytes, displays the same pharmacological character-istics as those reported in OHCs (Elgoyhen, Johnson, Boulter, Vetter, & Heinemann, 1994). Receptor activation allows a calcium influx (Blanchet, Erostegui, Sugasawa, & Dulon, 1996; Doi & Ohmori, 1993; Erostegui, Norris, & Bobbin, 1994; Housley & Ashmore, 1991; Nenov, Norris, & Bobbin, 1996a) followed by secondary events, occurring on two different time scales. The "fast response," taking milliseconds, is associated with an outward K+ current that results in hyperpolariza-tion of the OHC membrane (Blanchet et al., 1996; Evans, 1996; Fuchs & Murrow, 1992; McNiven, Yuhas, & Fuchs, 1996; Nenov et al., 1996a, 1996b). The "slow response," which develops in ~20 seconds (Dallos et al., 1997; Sridhar et al., 1995), is likely produced by a second-mes-senger system. While efferent stimulation inhibits cochlear processing, ACh increases electromotility in isolated OHCs (Sziklai & Dallos, 1993; Sziklai, He, & Dallos, 1996). This increase is thought to reflect a decrease in cell stiffness (Dallos et al., 1997). The ACh effect is proba-bly related to an intracellular calcium-dependent phenomenon (Dallos et al., 1997; Sridhar et al., 1995). The apparent paradox of a generally inhibitory efferent effect and a facilitatory effect of ACh on isolated OHC motility may relate to a fundamental difference in the mechanics of isolated cells versus those of in vivo preparations (Kolston, 1999).

DISCOVERY OF MOTOR PROTEIN

OHC electromotility is the likely result of the concentrated action of a large number of independent molecular motors that are closely asso-ciated with the cell's basolateral membrane (Dallos, Evans, & Hallworth, 1991; Holley & Ashmore, 1988a; Huang & Santos-Sacchi,

1993), possibly the densely packed 10 nm particles (Forge, 1991; Gulley & Reese, 1977) seen therein. Based on similarities between the cortical structure of erythrocytes and OHCs, it has been proposed that the motor molecule is a modified anion exchanger (Kalinec & Kachar, 1993; Knipper et al., 1995). Because their shallow voltage dependence matches that of charge movement in OHCs, transporters, as opposed to modified voltage-dependent channels, have been favored as likely candidates (Ashmore, 1992). A recent suggestion is that the motor is related to a fructose transporter, GLUT5 (Géléoc, Casalotti, Forge, & Ashcroft, 1999). However, until our work (Zheng et al., 2000), the molecular identity of the motor protein was unknown.

METHOD

There were two difficulties to our molecular approach to identify the OHC sensor-motor protein (Figure 1–6): first, isolation of cDNA from very small amounts of biological material, and second, recognition of the candidate motor protein cDNA among the isolated unknown genes. Isolation of a sufficient number of OHCs is a fairly routine task. Obtaining comparable numbers of IHCs, however, required some modification of techniques (He, Zheng, Edge, & Dallos, 2000). We were able to isolate mRNA from approximately 1,000 OHCs and 1,000 IHCs and used RT PCR amplification to obtain OHC and IHC cDNA pools. It was reasonable to expect that gene expression related to mechanoelectric transduction and genomic, metabolic, and structural functions would be shared by the two types of hair cell. Therefore, we applied a suppression subtractive hybridization PCR procedure to amplify and enrich the OHC cDNA pool for uniquely expressed gene products (Diatchenko et al., 1996).

Approximately 1,300 fragment clones were screened with four cDNA pools (OHC-IHC, IHC-OHC, OHC unsubtracted, and IHC unsubtracted) to identify differentially expressing clones. Once false positives were excluded, 487 clones were identified as differentially expressing, and of these the most promising 108 were sequenced. Because of duplicates, these 108 sequences identified 50 unique cDNA fragments. Eighteen of the clones had sequences highly similar to known proteins, while 32 were thought to be unique in that there were no obvious homologous sequences in the genetic database. Eleven of the 32 clones had apparent open reading frames. *Prestin* was one of the 11 candidate clones whose differential expression was most consistent

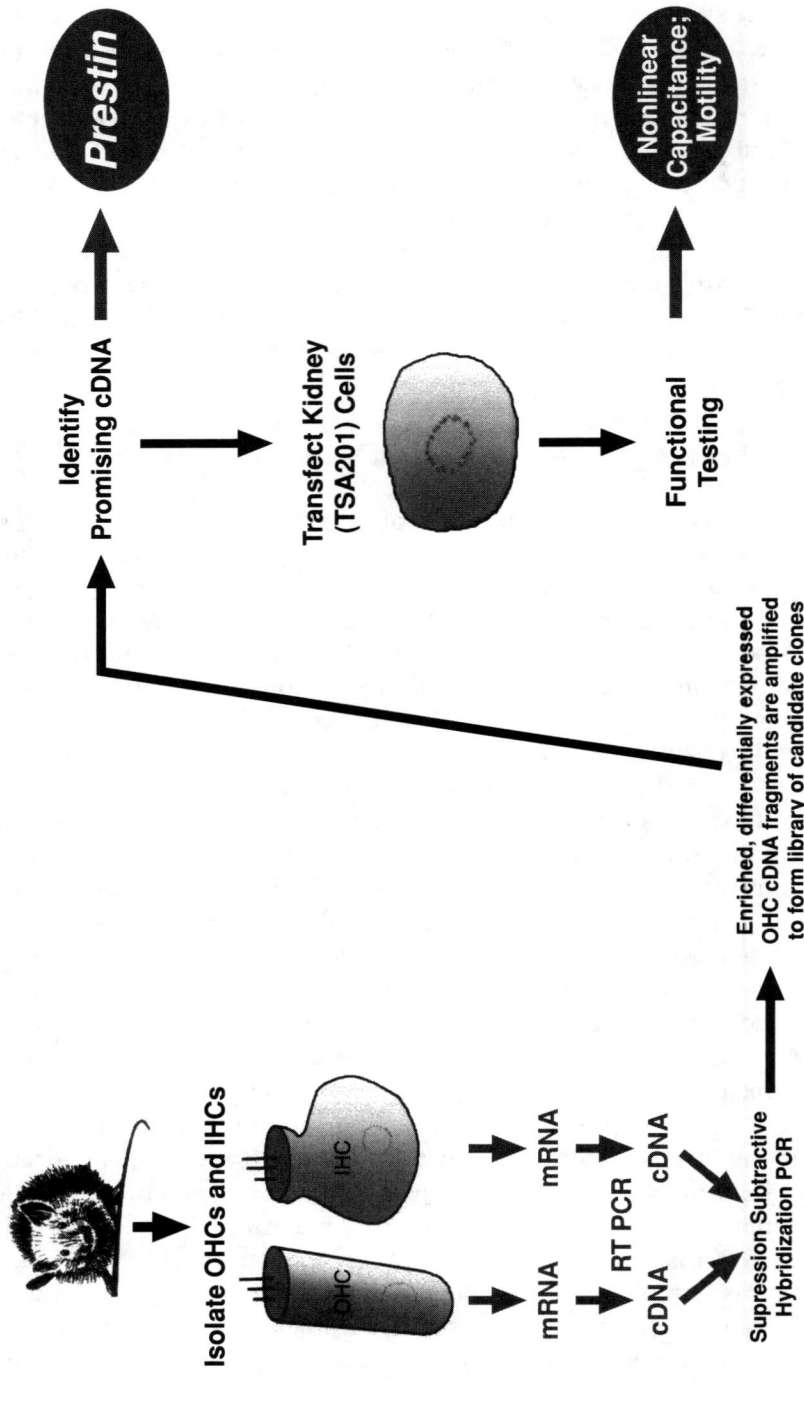

Figure 1–6. Schema of the approach to identifying the outer hair cell motor protein and its functional testing.

14

with our assumptions about the motor protein. Using a *PRES* cDNA *Rsal* fragment as a probe, we subsequently isolated the full-length cDNA *PRES* clone from a Xgtl 1 gerbil adult cochlea library (provided by Dr. Bradley Schulte). *Prestin* encodes a 744 amino acid protein, prestin. A computer search with the *PRES* sequence revealed that about one third of the human *PRES* gene has been already sequenced as part of the human chromosome 7 effort. The amino acid homology between human and gerbil prestin is 98%.

Analysis of the prestin sequence revealed that its highest homology was to members of a family of anion/sulfate transport proteins. The protein prestin (744 amino acids; 81.4 kDa) is hydrophobic, with −50% nonpolar residues. Computer modeling of the amino acid sequence produces ambiguous results as to the number and location of transmembrane regions and cannot predict the topology of the amino and carboxy termini in relation to the membrane. Antibodies are now available against epitopes in the N- and C-termini. It has been demonstrated that either antibody recognizes the protein only if the outer hair cells are permeabilized (N-terminus: Zheng et al., 2000; C-terminus: Belyantseva et al., 2000). Consequently, we now know that both termini are cytoplasmic. This knowledge reduces the topographic description of the protein to having either 10 or 12 transmembrane domains. Prestin shows high homology in the sulfate transport region, a highly conserved domain found in homologs in organisms as distant as yeast, *C. elegans,* and plants. However, both human and gerbil prestin differ from the consensus sequence at three positions. Consequently, while prestin appears related to sulfate transporters, these differences in the conserved region suggest that the protein may have distinct properties. It is now known that when expressed in frog oocyte, prestin does not function as an anion transporter (L. Kamiski, personal communication, April 1, 2000).

To test the sensor-motor function of prestin, voltage-dependent charge movement (Ashmore, 1989; Santos-Sacchi, 1991) was measured from human embryonic kidney (TSA201) cells after transient transfection of unmodified, native *PRES* cDNA. A second plasmid (pEGFP-N2) containing the green fluorescent protein (GFP) cDNA was used as an independent marker for successful transfection of the cells. In experiments conducted on cells co-transfected with prestin and GFP cDNA, transient capacitive currents were obtained from 91.8% of the GFP positive cells (45 out of 49). In contrast, untransfected cells ($n = 20$) or cells transfected with only the control plasmid ($n = 28$) had no measurable nonlinear capacitance. The numerical values that characterize the charge movement are similar to those obtained for OHCs (Huang & Santos-Sacchi, 1993). The maximum charge and charge density are less in the transfected cells even though the linear capacitance is about the same as that of an average OHC. In OHCs, nonlinear capacitive current and electromotility can be reversibly blocked by sodium salicylate (Kakehata & Santos-Sacchi, 1996; Shehata, Brownell, & Dieler, 1991; Tunstall, Galer, & Ashmore, 1995). As further evidence that transient currents stem from the transfected motor protein, salicylate was locally applied to cells that had been shown to present charge movement. Sodium salicylate significantly reduced the transient currents.

OHCs are efficient producers of axial motility because of their cylindrical shape. Fast mechanical effects occur at constant cell volume and are generally assumed to be the result of a change in cell surface area, due to the aggregate conformational shape changes of large numbers of motor proteins (Holley & Ashmore, 1988a; Kalinec et al., 1992). A spherical cell cannot change its surface area while its volume remains constant, whereas a cylindrical cell could (Adachi & Iwasa, 1999). In order that the generally spherical TSA201 cells may produce measurable motility, we distorted them to alter their shape by drawing them into a suction pipette. In spite of these difficulties, we succeeded in demonstrating electromotility in 7 of 31 cells tested. Sodium salicylate produced a reversible decrease in the electromotile response, just as it does in OHCs. Thus, we have now identified the gene that codes for a specialized motor protein that produces electromechanical action when expressed in cells that in their native form do not show this phenomenon.

Acknowledgment: This work was supported by the National Institute of Deafness and other Communication Disorders (NIDCD), the McKnight Foundation, and the American Hearing Research Foundation.

REFERENCES

Adachi, M., & Iwasa, K. H. (1999). Electrically driven motor in the outer hair cell: Effect of a mechanical constraint. *Proceedings of the National Academy of Sciences of the USA, 96,* 7244–7249.

Ashmore, J. F. (1987). A fast motile response in guinea-pig outer hair cells: The cellular basis of the cochlear amplifier. *Journal of Physiology (London), 388,* 323–347.

Ashmore, J. F. (1989). Transductor motor coupling in cochlear outer hair cells. In J. P. Wilson & D. T. Kemp (Eds.), *Mechanisms of hearing* (pp. 107–113). New York: Plenum Press.

Ashmore, J. F. (1992). Mammalian hearing and the cellular mechanisms of the cochlear amplifer. In D. P. Corey & S. D. Roper (Eds.), *Sensory transduction* (pp. 396–412). New York: Rockefeller University Press.

Assad, T. A., Hacohen, N., & Corev, D. P. (1989). Voltage dependence of adaptation and active bundle movement in bullfrog saccular hair cells. *Proceedings of the National Academy of Sciences of the USA, 86*, 2918–2922.

Békésy, G. V. (1960). *Experiments in hearing.* New York: McGraw-Hill.

Benser, M. E., Marquis, R. E., & Hudspeth, A. J. (1996). Rapid active hair bundle movements in hair cells from the bullfrog's sacculus. *Journal of Neuroscience, 16*(18), 5629–5643.

Billone, M. C., & Raynor, S. (1973). Transmission of radial shear forces to cochlear hair cells. *Journal of the Acoustical Society of America, 54*, 1143–1156.

Blanchet, C., Erostegui, C., Sugasawa, M., & Dulon, D. (1996). Acetylcholine-induced potassium current of guinea pig outer hair cells: Its dependence on a calcium influx through nicotinic-like receptors. *Journal of Neuroscience, 16*, 2574–2584.

Brown, M. C., & Nuttall, A. L. (1984). Efferent control of cochlear inner hair cells responses in the guinea-pig. *Journal of Physiology, 354*, 625–646.

Brownell, W. E. (1983). Observations on a motile response in isolated outer hair cells. In W. R. Webster & L. M. Aitkin (Eds.), *Mechanisms of hearing* (pp. 5–10). Clayton, Australia: Monash University Press.

Brownell, W. E., Bader, C. R., Bertrand, D., & deRibaupierre, Y. (1985). Evoked mechanical responses of isolated cochlear outer hair cells. *Science, 227*, 194–196.

Camalet, D., Duke, T., Julicher, F., & Prost, J. (2000). Auditory sensitivity provided by self–tuned critical oscillations of hair cells. *Proceedings of the National Academy of Sciences of the USA, 97*, 3183–3188.

Choe, T., Magnasco, M. O., & Hudspeth, A. J. (1998). A model for amplification of hair–bundle motion by cyclical binding of Ca2+ to mechanoelectrical-transduction channels. *Proceedings of the National Academy of Sciences of the USA, 95*, 15321–15326

Corti, A. (1851). Recherches sur l'organe de l'ouie des mammiferes. *Zuricher Zeitschrift fur Wissenschaft Zoologie, 3*, 109–169.

Crawford, A. C., & Fettiplace, R. (1985). The mechanical properties of ciliary bundles of turtle cochlear hair cells. *Journal of Physiology (London), 364*, 359–379.

Dallos, P. (1973). Cochlear potentials and cochlear mechanics. In A. Moller (Ed.), *Basic mechanisms in hearing* (pp. 335–372). New York: Academic Press.

Dallos, P. (1985). The role of outer hair cells in cochlear function. In M. J. Correia & A. A. Perachio (Eds.), *Contemporary sensory neurobiology* (pp. 207–230). New York: Alan R. Liss.

Dallos, P. (1988). Cochlear neurobiology: Some key experiments and concepts of the past two decades. In G. M. Edelman, E. W. Gall, & M. W. Cowan (Eds.), *Functions of the auditory system* (pp. 153–188). New York: Wiley.

Dallos, P. (1992). The active cochlea. *Journal of Neuroscience, 12,* 4575–4585.

Dallos, P., Billone, M. C., Durrant, J. D., Wang, C. Y., & Raynor, S. (1972). Cochlear inner and outer hair cells: Functional differences. *Science, 177,* 356–358.

Dallos, P., & Cheatham, M. A. (1976). Production of cochlear potentials by inner and outer hair cells. *Journal of the Acoustical Society of America, 60,* 510–512.

Dallos, P., & Evans, B. N. (1995). High-frequency motility of outer hair cells and the cochlear amplifier. *Science, 267,* 2006–2009.

Dallos, P., Evans, B. N., & Hallworth, R. (1991). Nature of the motor element in electrokinetic shape changes of cochlear outer hair cells. *Nature, 350,* 155–157.

Dallos, P., & Harris, D. (1978). Properties of auditory nerve responses in absence of outer hair cells. *Journal of Neurophysiology, 41,* 365–383.

Dallos, P., Harris, D. M., Relkin, E., & Cheatham, M. A. (1980). Two-tone suppression and intermodulation distortion in the cochlea: Effect of outer hair cell lesions. In G. van den Brink & F. A. Bilsen (Eds.), *Psychophysical, physiological and behavioral studies in hearing* (pp. 242–249). Delft, The Netherlands: Delft University Press.

Dallos, P., He, D. Z. Z., Sziklai, I., Lin, X., Mehta, S., & Evans, B. N. (1997). Acetylcholine, outer hair cell electromotility, and the cochlear amplifier. *Journal of Neuroscience, 15,* 2212–2226.

Dallos, P., Schoeny, Z. G., Worthington, D. W., & Cheatham, M. A. (1969). Cochlear distortion: Effect of direct-current polarization. *Science, 164,* 449–451.

Dallos P., & Wang, C. Y. (1974). Bioelectric correlates of kanamycin intoxication. *Audiology, 12,* 277–289.

Davis, H. (1959). An interpretation of the mechanical detector action of the cochlea. *Annals of Otology, Rhinology, and Laryngology, 68,* 665–674.

Davis, H. (1960). Mechanism of excitation of auditory and nerve impulses. In G. L. Rasmussen & W. Windle (Eds.), *Neural mechanisms of the auditory and vestibular systems* (pp. 21–39). Springfield, IL: Charles C. Thomas.

Davis, H., Deatherage, B. H., Rosenblut, B., Fernandez, C., Kimura, R., & Smith, C. A. (1958). Modification of cochlear potentials produced by streptomycin poisoning and extensive venous obstruction. *Laryngoscope, 68,* 596–627.

Diatchenko, L., Lau, Y. F. C., Campbell, A. P., Chechik, A., Mogadam, F., Huang, B., Lukyanoc, S., Gurskaya, D., Sverdlov, E. D., & Siebert, P. D. (1996). Suppression subtractive hybridization: A method for generating differentially regulated or tissue-specific cDNA probes and libraries. *Proceedings of the National Academy of Sciences of the USA, 93,* 6025–6030.

Doi, T., & Ohmori, H. (1993). Acetylcholine increases intracellular Ca+ concentration and hyperpolarizes the guinea–pig outer hair cell. *Hearing Research, 67,* 179–188.

Eguiluz, V. M., Ospeck, M., Choe, Y., Hudspeth, A. J., & Magnasco, M. O. (2000). Essential nonlinearities in hearing. *Physical Review Letters, 84,* 5232–5235.

Elgoyhen, A. B., Johnson, D. S., Boulter, J., Vetter, D. E., & Heinemann, S. (1994). Alpha 9: An acetylcholine receptor with novel pharmacological properties expressed in rat cochlear hair cells. *Cell, 79,* 705–715.

Engström, H. (1958). Structure and intervention of the inner ear sensory epithelia. *International Review of Cytology, 7,* 535–585.

Engström, H., Ades, H. W., & Hawkins, J. E., Jr. (1962). Structure and functions of the sensory hairs of the inner hair cell. *Journal of the Acoustical Society of America, 34,* 1356–1363.

Erostegui, C., Norris, C. H., & Bobbin, R. P. (1994). Acetylcholine activates a K+ conductance permeable to Cs+ in guinea pig outer hair cells. *Hearing Research, 74,* 135–147.

Evans, B. N., & Dallos, P. (1993). Stereocilia displacement induced somatic motility of cochlear outer hair cells. *Proceedings of the National Academy of Sciences of the USA, 90,* 8347–9351.

Evans, B. N., Dallos, P., & Hallworth, R. (1989). Assymetrics in motile responses of outer hair cells in simulated in vivo conditions. In J. P. Wilson & D. T. Kemp (Eds.), *Cochlear mechanisms* (pp. 205–206). London: Plenum Press.

Evans, B. N., Hallworth, R., & Dallos, P. (1991). Outer hair cell electromobility: The sensitivity and vulnerability of the DC component. *Hearing Research, 52,* 288–304.

Evans, E. F., & Wilson, J. P. (1973). The frequency selectivity of the cochlea. In A. Moller (Ed.), *Basic mechanisms in hearing* (pp. 519–554). London: Academic Press.

Evans, M. G. (1996). Acetylcholine activates two currents in guinea pig outer hair cells. *Journal of Physiology (London), 491,* 563–578.

Eybalin, M. (1993). Neurotransmitters and neuromodulators of the mammalian cochlea. *Physiological Reviews, 73,* 309–373.

Forge, A. (1991). Structural features of the lateral walls in mammalian cochlear outer hair cells. *Cell Tissue Research, 265,* 473–483.

Frank, G., Hemmert, W., & Gummer, A. W. (1999). Limiting dynamics of high-frequency electromechanical transduction of outer hair cells. *Proceedings of the National Academy of Sciences of the USA, 96,* 4420–4425.

Fuchs, P. A., & Murrow, B. W. (1992). Cholinergic inhibition of short (outer) hair cells of the chick's cochlea. *Journal of Neuroscience, 12,* 800–809.

Galambos, R. (1956). Suppression of auditory nerve activity by stimulation of efferent fibers to cochlea. *Journal of Neurophysiology, 19,* 424–437.

Gale, J. E., & Ashmore, J. F. (1997). An intrinsic frequency limit to the cochlear amplifier. *Nature, 389,* 63–66.

Géléoc, G. S. G., Casalotti, S. O., Forge, A., & Ashcroft, J. F. (1999). A sugar transporter as a candidate for the outer hair cell motor. *Nature Neuroscience, 2,* 713–719.

Gitter, A. H., Rudert, M., & Zenner, H. P. (1993). Forces involved in length changes of cochlear outer hair cells. *Pfugers Archives, 424,* 9–14.

Goldstein, J. L. (1967). Auditory nonlinearity. *Journal of the Acoustical Society of America, 41,* 676–689.

Guinan, J. J. (1996). Physiology of olivocochlear efferents. In P. Dallos, A. Popper, & R. R. Fay (Eds.), *The cochlea* (pp. 435–502). New York: Springer-Verlag.

Guinan, J. J., & Peake, W. T. (1967). Middle-ear characteristics of anesthetized cats. *Journal of the Acoustical Society of America, 41,* 1237–1261.

Gulley, R. L., & Reese, T. S. (1977). Regional specialization of the hair cell plasmalemma in the organ of Corti. *Anatomical Research, 189,* 109–123.

Guth, P. S., & Norris, C. H. (1996). The hair cell acetylcholine receptors: A synthesis. *Hearing Research, 98,* 1–8.

Hallworth, R. (1995). Passive compliance and active force generation in the guinea pig outer hair cell. *Journal of Neurophysiology, 74,* 2319–2328.

He, D. Z. Z., & Dallos, P. (1999). Somatic stiffness of cochlear outer hair cells is voltage dependent. *Proceedings of the National Academy of Sciences of the USA, 96,* 8223–8228.

He, D. Z. Z., & Dallos, P. (2000). Properties of voltage-dependent somatic stiffness of cochlear outer hair cells. *JARO: Journal of the Association for Research in Otolaryngology, 1,* 64–81.

He, D. Z. Z., Zheng, J., Edge, R., & Dallos, P. (2000). Isolation of cochlear inner hair cells. *Hearing Research, 145,* 156–160.

Hensen, V. (1863). Zur morphlogie der schnecke des menschen und der Saugetiere. *Zuricher Zeitschrift fur Wissenschaft Zoologie, 13,* 481–512.

Holley, M. C. (1996). Outer hair cell motility. In P. Dallos, A. Popper, & R. Fay (Eds.), *The cochlea* (pp. 386–434). New York: Springer-Verlag.

Holley, M. C., & Ashmore, J. F. (1988a). On the mechanism of a high frequency force generator in outer hair cells isolated from the guinea pig cochlea. *Proceedings of the Royal Society of London Biological Science, 232,* 413–429.

Holley, M. C., & Ashmore, J. F. (1988b). A cytoskeletal spring in cochlear outer hair cells. *Nature, 335,* 635–637.

Housley, G. D., & Ashmore, J. F. (1991). Direct measurement of the action of acetylcholine on isolated outer hair cells of the guinea pig cochlea. *Proceedings of the Royal Society of London Biological Science, 244,* 161–167.

Hu, X. T., Evans, B. N., He, D. Z. Z., & Dallos, P. (1994). Distortion products in electromotile responses of isolated outer hair cells. *Abstracts of the Midwinter Research Meeting of the Association for Research in Otolaryngology, 17,* 125.

Huang, G., & Santos-Sacchi, J. (1993). Mapping the distribution of the outer hair cell motility voltage sensor by electrical amputation. *Biophysiology Journal, 65,* 2228–2236.

Hudspeth, A. J. (1989). How the ear's works work. *Nature, 341,* 397–404.

Hudspeth, A. J. (1997). Mechanical amplification of stimuli by hair cells. *Current Opinions in Neurobiology, 7,* 480–486.

Iwasa, K. H., & Adachi, M. (1997). Force generation in the outer hair cell of the cochlea. *Biophysiology Journal, 73,* 546–555.

Iwasa, K. H., & Kachar, B. (1989). Fast in vitro movement of outer hair cells in an external electric field: Effect of digitonin, a membrane permeabilizing agent. *Hearing Research, 40,* 247–254.

Kachar, B., Brownell, W. E., Altschuler, R, & Fex, J. (1986). Electrokinetic shape changes of cochlear outer hair cells. *Nature, 322,* 365–368.

Kakehata, S., & Santos-Sacchi, J. (1996). Effects of salicylate and lanthanides on outer hair cell motility and associated gating charge. *Journal of Neuroscience, 16,* 4881–4889.

Kalinec, F., Holley, M. C., Iwasa, K., Lim, D. J., & Kachar, B. (1992). A membrane–based force generation mechanism in auditory sensory cells. *Proceedings of the National Academy of Sciences of the USA, 89,* 8671–8675.

Kalinec, F., & Kachar, B. (1993). Inhibition of outer hair cell electromotility by sulfhydryl specific reagents. *Neuroscience Letters, 157,* 231–234.

Kemp, D. T. (1978). Stimulated acoustic emissions from within the human auditory system. *Journal of the Acoustical Society of America, 64,* 1386–1391.

Kemp, D. T. (1979). Evidence of mechanical nonlinearity and frequency selective wave amplification in the cochlea. *Archives of Otolaryngology—Head and Neck Surgery, 224,* 37–45.

Khanna, S. M., & Leonard, D. G. B. (1982). Basilar membrane tuning in the cat cochlea. *Science, 215,* 305–306.

Kiang, N. Y. S., Moxon, E. C., & Levine, R. A. (1970). Auditory–nerve activity in cats with normal and abnormal cochleas. In G. E. W. Wolstenholme & J. Knight (Eds.), *Sensorineural hearing loss* (pp. 241–268). CIBA Foundation Symposium. London: Churchill.

Kim, D. O. (1986). Active and nonlinear cochlear biomechanics and the role of the outer hair cell sub-system in the mammalian auditory system. *Hearing Research, 22,* 105–114.

Kimura, R. S. (1966). Frequency tuning of basilar membrane and auditory nerve fibers in the same cochleae. *Acta Otolaryngologica, 61,* 55–72.

Knipper, M., Zimmerman, U., Kopschall, I., Rohbock, K., Jungling, S., & Zenner, H. P. (1995). Immunological identification of candidate proteins involved in regulating active shape changes of outer hair cells. *Hearing Research, 86,* 100–110.

Kohllöffel, L. U. E. (1972). A study of basilar membrane vibrations. Part II: The vibratory amplitude and phase pattern along the basilar membrane. *Acoustica, 27,* 66–81.

Kolston, P. J. (1999). Comparing in vitro, in situ, and in vivo experimental data in a three-dimensional model of mammalian cochlear mechanics. *Proceedings of the National Academy of Sciences of the USA, 96,* 3676–3681.

Köppl, C. (1995). Otoacoustic emissions as an indicator for active cochlear mechanics: A primitive property of vertebrate auditory organs. In G. A. Manley, G. M. Klump, C. Koppl, H. Fastl, & H. Oeckinghaus (Eds.), *Advances in hearing research* (pp. 207–216). Singapore: World Scientific Press.

Lim, D. J. (1972). Fine morphology of the tectorial membrane: Its relationship to the organ of Corti. *Archives of Otolaryngology—Head and Neck Surgery, 96,* 199–215.

Lindemann, H. H., Ades, H. W., Bredberg, G., & Engström, H. (1971). The sensory hairs and the tectorial membrane in the development of the cat's organ of Corti: A scanning electron microscope study. *Acta Otolaryngologica, 72,* 229–242.

Lynn, P. A., & Sayers, B. (1970). Cochlear innervation, signal processing, and their relation to auditory time-intensity effects. *Journal of the Acoustical Society of America, 47,* 525–533.

Mammano, F., & Ashmore, J. F. (1993). Reverse transduction measured in the isolated cochlea by laser Michelson interferometry. *Nature, 365,* 838–841.

Manley, G. A., & Köppl, C. (1998). Phylogenetic development of the cochlea and its innervation. *Current Opinions in Neurobiology, 8,* 468–474.

Martin, P., & Hudspeth, A. J. (1999). Active hair-bundle movements can amplify a hair cell's response to oscillatory mechanical stimuli. *Proceedings of the National Academy of Sciences of the USA, 96,* 14306–14311.

McNiven, A. I., Yuhas, W. A., & Fuchs, P. A. (1996). Ionic dependence and agonist preference of an acetylcholine receptor in hair cells. *Auditory Neuroscience, 2,* 63–77.

Mountain, D. C. (1980). Changes in endolymphatic potential and crossed olivocochlear bundle stimulation alter cochlear mechanics. *Science, 210,* 71–72.

Mountain, D. C., & Hubbard, A. E. (1994). A piezoelectric model of outer hair cell function. *Journal of the Acoustical Society of America, 95,* 350–354.

Mountain, D. C., Hubbard, A. E., & McMullen, T. A. (1983). Electromechanical processes in the cochlea. In E. deBoer & M. Viergever (Eds.), *Mechanics of hearing* (pp. 119–126). Delft, The Netherlands: Delft University Press.

Murugasu, E., & Russell, I. J. (1996). The effect of efferent stimulation of basilar membrane displacement in the basal turn of the guinea pig cochlea. *Journal of Neuroscience, 16,* 325–332.

Narayan, S. S., Temchin, A. N., Recio, A., & Ruggero, M. A. (1998). Frequency tuning of basilar membrane and auditory nerve fibers in the same cochlea. *Science, 282,* 1882–1884.

Nenov, A. P., Norris, C, & Bobbin, R. P. (1996a). Acetycholine response in guinea pig outer hair cells; Part 1: Properties of the response. *Hearing Research, 101,* 132–148.

Nenov, A. P., Norris, C, & Bobbin, R. P. (1996b).). Acetycholine response in guinea pig outer hair cells; Part 2: Activation of a small conductance Ca(2+)-activated K+ channel. *Hearing Research, 101,* 149–172.

Nuttall, A. L., & Dolan, D. F. (1993). Intermodulation distortion (F2–F1) in inner hair cell and basilar membrane responses. *Journal of the Acoustical Society of America, 93,* 2061–2068.

Oghalai, J. S., Patel, A. A., Nakagawa, T., & Brownell, W. E. (1998). Fluorescence-imaged microdeformation of the outer hair cell lateral wall. *Journal of Neuroscience, 18,* 48–58.

Patuzzi, R. (1996). Cochlear micromechanics and macromechanics. In P. Dallos, A. Popper, & R. Fay (Eds.), *The cochlea* (pp. 186–257). New York: Springer-Verlag.

Probst, R. (1990). Otoacoustic emissions: An overview. In C. R. Pfaltz (Ed.), *New aspects of cochlear mechanics and inner ear pathophysiology* (pp. 1–91). (From *Advances in Otorhinolaryngology, 44.*)

Probst, R., Lonsbury-Martin, B. L., & Martin, G. K. (1991). A review of otoacoustic emissions. *Journal of the Acoustical Society of America, 89,* 2027–2067.

Rhode, W. S. (1971). Observation of the vibration of the basilar membrane in squirrel monkeys using the Mossbauer technique. *Journal of the Acoustical Society of America, 49,* 1218–1231.

Rhode, W. S. (1973). An investigation of postmortem cochlear mechanics using the Mossbauer technique. In A. R. Moller (Ed.), *Basic mechanisms of hearing* (pp. 49–67). New York: Academic Press.

Ricci, A. J., Crawford, A. C., & Fettiplace, R. (2000). Active hair bundle motion linked to fast transducer adaptation in auditory hair cells. *Journal of Neuroscience, 20,* 7131–7142.

Robles, L., Ruggero, M. A., & Rich, N. C. (1986). Basilar membrane mechanics at the base of the chinchilla cochlea. Part I: Input-output functions, tuning curves, and response phases. *Journal of the Acoustical Society of America, 80,* 1364–1374.

Ruggero, M. A., Rich, N. C., Recio, A., Narayan, S. S., & Robles, L. (1997). Basilar-membrane responses to tones at the base of the chinchilla cochlea. *Journal of the Acoustical Society of America, 101,* 2151–2163.

Russell, I. J., & Schauz, C. (1995). Salicylate ototoxicity: Effects on the stiffness and electromotility of outer hair cells isolated from the guinea pig cochlea. *Auditory Neuroscience, 1,* 309–319.

Ryan, A., & Dallos, P. (1975). Absence of cochlear outer hair cells: Effect on behavioral auditory threshold. *Nature, 253,* 44–46.

Santos-Sacchi, J. (1989). A symmetry in voltage-dependent movements of isolated outer hair cells from the organ of Corti. *Journal of Neuroscience, 9,* 2954–2962.

Santos-Sacchi, J. (1991). Reversible inhibition of voltage-dependent outer hair cell motility and capacitance. *Journal of Neuroscience, 11,* 3096–3110.

Santos-Sacchi, J. (1992). On the frequency limit and phase of outer hair cell motility: Effects of the membrane filter. *Journal of Neuroscience, 12,* 1906–1916.

Santos-Sacchi, J., & Dilger, J. P. (1988). Whole cell currents and mechanical responses of isolated outer hair cells. *Hearing Research, 35,* 143–150.

Schmiedt, R. A., Zwislocki, J. J., & Hamernik, R. P. (1980). Effects of hair cell lesions on responses of cochlear nerve fibers. Part 1: Lesions, tuning curves, two-tone inhibition, and responses to trapezoidal wave patterns. *Journal of Neurophysiology, 43,* 1367–1389.

Sellick, P. M., Patuzzi, R., & Johnstone, B. M. (1982). Measurement of basilar membrane motion in the guinea-pig using the Mossbauer technique. *Journal of the Acoustical Society of America, 72,* 131–141.

Shehata, W., Brownell, W. E., & Dieler, R. (1991). Effects of salicylate on shape, electromotility and membrane characteristics of isolated outer hair cells from guinea pig cochlea. *Acta Otolaryngologica (Stockholm), 111,* 707–718.

Siegel, J. H., & Kim, D. O. (1982). Efferent neural control of cochlear mechanics? Olivocochlear bundle stimulation affects cochlear biomechanical nonlinearity. *Hearing Research, 6,* 171–182.

Smith, C. A., & Sjöstrand, F. S. (1961a). Structure of the nerve endings on the external hair cells of the guinea pig cochlea as studied by serial sections. *Journal of Ultrastructure Research, 5,* 184–192.

Smith, C. A., & Sjöstrand, F. S. (1961b). Structure of the nerve endings on the external hair cells of the guinea pig cochlea as studied by serial sections. *Journal of Ultrastructure Research, 5,* 523–556.

Spoendlin, H. (1966). *The organization of the cochlear receptor.* Basel: Karger.

Spoendlin, H. (1969). Innervation patterns in the organ of Corti in the cat. *Acta Otolaryngologica, 67,* 239–254.

Sridhar, T. S., Liberman, M. C., Brown, M. C., & Sewell, W. F. (1995). A novel cholinergic "slow effect" of efferent stimulation on cochlear potentials in the guinea pig. *Journal of Neuroscience, 15,* 3667–3678.

Sziklai, I., & Dallos, P. (1993). Acetylcholine controls the gain of voltage-to-movement converter in isolated outer hair cells. *Acta Otolaryngologica (Stockholm), 113,* 326–329.

Sziklai, I., He, D. Z. Z., & Dallos, P. (1996). Effect of acetylcholine and GABA on the transfer function of electromotility in isolated outer hair cells. *Hearing Research, 95,* 87–99.

Tolomeo, J. A., Steele, C. R., & Holley, M. C. (1996). Mechanical properties of the lateral cortex of mammalian auditory outer hair cells. *Biophysiological Journal, 71,* 421–429.

Tunstall, M. J., Gale, L. E., & Ashmore, J. F. (1995). Action of salicylate on membrane capacitance of outer hair cells from the guinea-pig cochlea. *Journal of Physiology (London), 485,* 739–752.

Ulfendahl, M., Flock, A. A. (1998). Outer hair cells provide active tuning in the organ of Corti. *News in Physiological Sciences, 13,* 107–111.

Van Dijk, P., Manley, G. A., & Gallo, I. (1998). Correlated amplitude fluctuations of spontaneous otoacoustic emissions in six lizard species. *Journal of the Acoustical Society of America, 104,* 1559–1564.

Wilson, J. P. (1980). Evidence for cochlear origin for acoustic re-emissions, threshold fine–structure and tonal tinnitus. *Hearing Research, 2,* 233–252.

Xue, Z., Shan, X., Lapeyre, B., & Melese, T. (1993). The amino terminus of mammalian nucleolin specifically recognizes SV40 T-antigen type nuclear localization sequences. *European Journal of Cell Biology, 62*(1), 13–21.

Zheng, J., Shen, W., He, D. Z. Z., Long, K., Madison, L. D., & Dallos, P. (2000). Prestin is the motor protein of cochlear outer hair cells. *Nature, 405,* 149–155.

Zwislocki, J. J. (1974). A possible neuro-mechanical sound analysis in the cochlea. *Acustica, 31,* 354–359.

Zwislocki, J. J. (1977). Further indirect evidence for interaction between cochlear inner and outer hair cells. In E. F. Evans & J. P. Wilson (Eds.), *Psychophysics and physiology of hearing* (pp. 125–135). London: Academic Press.

2

On the Origins of the Outer Hair Cell Electromotility

W. E. Brownell, PhD

Bobby R. Alford Department of Otorhinolaryngology
and Communicative Sciences
Baylor College of Medicine
Houston, Texas

When outer hair cell electromotility was discovered it was an obvious candidate for the source of mechanical energy required for the mammalian cochlear amplifier. While outer hair cell electromotility provided answers for the hearing sciences it was in the uncomfortable position of appearing to be an isolated biological phenomenon. The source of energy appeared to be a previously unknown membrane-based force transduction mechanism. Yet the process of evolution is a conservative process in which existing mechanisms and molecules undergo slight changes to improve performance. This chapter examines the evolutionary forces that led to outer hair cell electromotility. It observes that hair cells are terminally differentiated epithelial cells whose apical and basal poles differ structurally and functionally, and it considers the implications of motile mechanisms in the apical pole. The structural and functional similarities between the apical pole and the outer hair cell lateral wall are then described. The remarkable structural similarities between the lateral wall and the cell wall of gliding bacteria are then presented, raising the possibility that the outer hair cell is using an ancient mechanism for cell motility based on highly curved membranes. If membrane curvature contributes to mechanical force generation it may play a role in the fusion of highly curved synaptic vesicles to presynaptic membranes, and this brings the chapter to its final section on the hair cell's basal pole.

THE APICAL POLE:
MECHANOELECTRICAL TRANSDUCTION

Hair cells are named for the bundle of enlarged microvilli referred to as stereocilia at their apical pole. The bundle supports mechanoelectrical transduction: deflection of the bundle modulates the flow of ions through specialized ion channels located near thin, extracellular, filamentous tip-links that connect the tops of all but the tallest stereocilia with their next tallest neighbor (Kachar, Parakkal, Kurc, Zhao, & Gillespie, 2000; Osborne, Comis, & Pickles, 1984; Pickles, Comis, & Osborne, 1984). Modulation of ionic flux results in hair cell receptor potentials. The kinetics of the mechanoelectrical transduction channels exceed those required for the behavioral frequency limits of the animal (Corey & Hudspeth, 1979).

High-frequency sounds contain information important for survival (such as determining the location of a sound in space), creating a selection pressure to increase the ear's frequency range. Because vertebrate-hearing organs are fluid-filled, viscous damping limits the highest frequency at which vertebrate sensory structures can vibrate. Middle ear structures have evolved to transmit an ever-broader range of frequencies (Allman, 1999), and the enhanced transmission had to be matched by inner ear strategies to overcome viscous damping if the organism was to hear the higher frequencies. A general class of electromechanical force transduction strategies appears to have come about. Some are located in the stereocilia and use adenosine triphosphate (ATP) and calcium in a manner similar to the cell motility mechanisms found in other eukaryotic cells. The membrane-based motor mechanism of the outer hair cell appeared later with the advent of mammals and is independent of cellular stores of ATP and calcium.

THE APICAL POLE:
ELECTROMECHANICAL TRANSDUCTION

Gold (1948) realized that the inner ear's fluid environment would degrade mechanical tuning and proposed that the upper frequency limit might be extended by a mechanism whereby mechanical energy is pumped into its vibrating structures. The positive feedback would effectively produce a negative damping force and counteract viscous damping. The process refines the band-pass filtering of cochlear vibrations, and because viscous damping is proportional to frequency the requirement for feedback becomes more demanding at high frequencies (Brownell, Spector, Raphael, & Popel, 2001). Davis (1983) coined the term "cochlear amplifier" for this mechanism after compelling evidence for its existence in the mammalian cochlea was obtained. A form of the cochlear amplifier is likely to be found throughout the vertebrate kingdom because all must deal with a fluid-filled inner ear. Manley (2000) has reviewed the evidence for the existence of a cochlear amplifier in vertebrates other than mammals. He points out that features of the cochlear amplifier (high sensitivity and frequency selectivity of hearing; compressive nonlinearities in afferent fiber rate-level functions; and otoacoustic emissions) are present in nonmammals and argues that the cochlear amplifier appears throughout the vertebrate family tree. While outer hair cell electromotility is the likely cochlear amplifier in mammals it is possible that the cochlear amplifier is associated with stereocilia bundle motility in nonmammals.

Mechanoelectric transduction channels in the stereocilia of many if not all hair cells have the ability to change their conductance with prolonged stimulus. The change is referred to as adaptation, and it is an electromechanical event. A sustained ionic flux (involving calcium) results in a change in the mechanical force acting on the mechanoelectrical transduction channel. Adaptation is particularly important for the vestibular system where a sustained bundle displacement comes about from a maintained head tilt. The sensitivity of the organ would be compromised in the absence of adaptation. Two types of calcium-dependent adaptation mechanisms have been identified; one with longer (> 10 ms) and the other with shorter (< 1 ms) time constants (Eatock, 2000; Ricci, Crawford, & Fettiplace, 2000). The molecular mechanism underlying both forms of adaptation is not known. The adaptation of hair cell receptor potentials has been linked with active mechanical movements of the stereocilia bundle (Choe, Magnasco, & Hudspeth, 1998; Crawford & Fettiplace, 1985; Denk & Webb, 1992; Howard & Hudspeth, 1987; Martin & Hudspeth, 1999; Ricci et al., 2000; Rusch & Thurm, 1990). Since an electromechanical force transduction mechanism exists in the stereocilia bundle it is possible that the bundle is the non-mammalian cochlear amplifier (Hudspeth, 1997). A stereocilia bundle locus for the cochlear amplifier is consistent with the large number of stereocilia per bundle (up to three times that of mammalian cochlear hair cells). A cochlear amplifier based on the stereocilia bundle may have been sufficient to provide negative damping at frequencies reaching the upper limit of reptiles (< 3 kHz) and birds (< 10 kHz). The mammalian cochlear amplifier is the outer hair cell and is based on a membrane motor mechanism that can reach frequencies approaching 100 kHz.

THE APICAL POLE: A TRILAMINATE STRUCTURE

The hair cell apical pole consists of three layers: (a) the plasma membrane; (b) a cytoskeletal matrix; and (c) the membranous canalicular reticulum (Figure 2–1). The plasma membrane follows the contours of the cytoskeletal matrix immediately beneath it. Stereocilia are organized around densely packed bundles of F-actin. These bundles have rootlets anchored in the hair cell's cuticular plate. The cuticular plate is composed of F-actin enriched by a number of other cytoskeletal proteins. The apical pole has a third layer immediately basal and

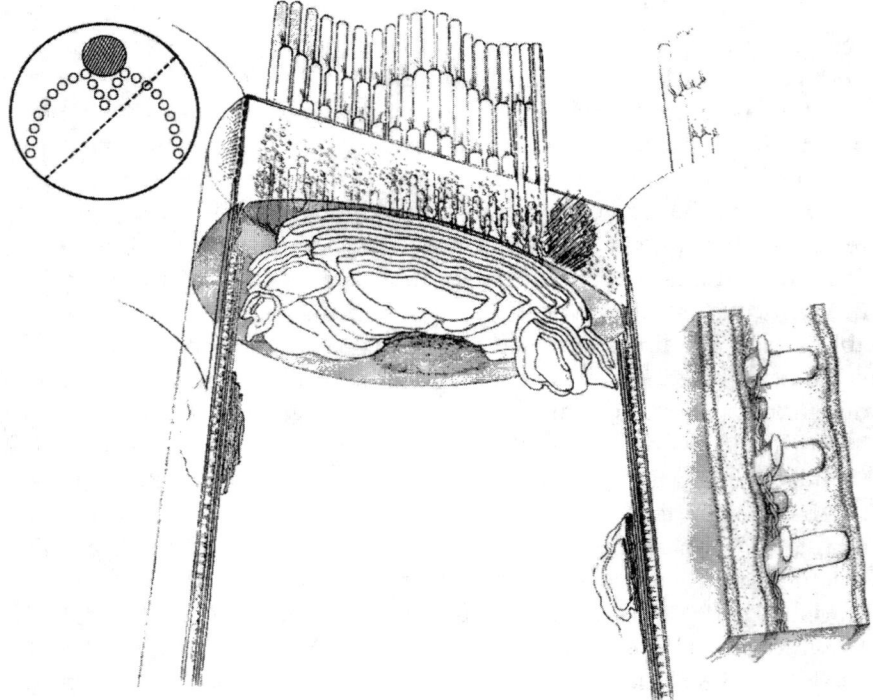

Figure 2–1. Three-layer organization in apical pole and the lateral wall of the cochlear outer hair cell. The outermost layer in both locations is the plasma membrane. The innermost layer is composed of a membrane-bound organelle called the canalicular reticulum in the apex and the subsurface cisterna in the lateral wall. In between the membranes is a cytoskeletal structure called the cuticular plate in the apex and the cortical lattice in the lateral wall. Insert at right shows a high-power rendering of the outer hair cell lateral wall. Insert at upper left is a view of the apical end showing the plane at which the outer hair cell has been opened.

adjacent to the cuticular plate. This layer consists of a complex of membranes called the canalicular reticulum, a structure that occurs in ion-transporting epithelia (Spicer, Thomopoulos, & Schulte, 1998). Membrane-bound organelles located in the hair cell apex have been noted in many early ultrastructural studies but it took postfixation with a ferrocyanide-osmium tetroxide solution (Spicer et al., 1998) to stabilize the canalicular reticulum membranes for ultrastructural studies. Their presence in living cells is revealed by fluorescent lipid markers (Oghalai, Patel, Nakagawa, & Brownell, 1998; Pollice & Brownell, 1993) revealing their role in organizing the apical pole. The three layers of the apical pole span a distance of ~1 μm. The apical pole is the likely precursor for a similar trilaminate organization in the outer hair cell lateral wall.

THE LATERAL WALL: A TRILAMINATE STRUCTURE

The trilaminate organization of the hair cell apical pole appears again in the outer hair cell (OHC) lateral wall (Figure 2–2). The OHC is a cylinder with a radius of ~4.5 μm. The three layers of its lateral wall form three axially concentric cylinders. The thickness of the lateral

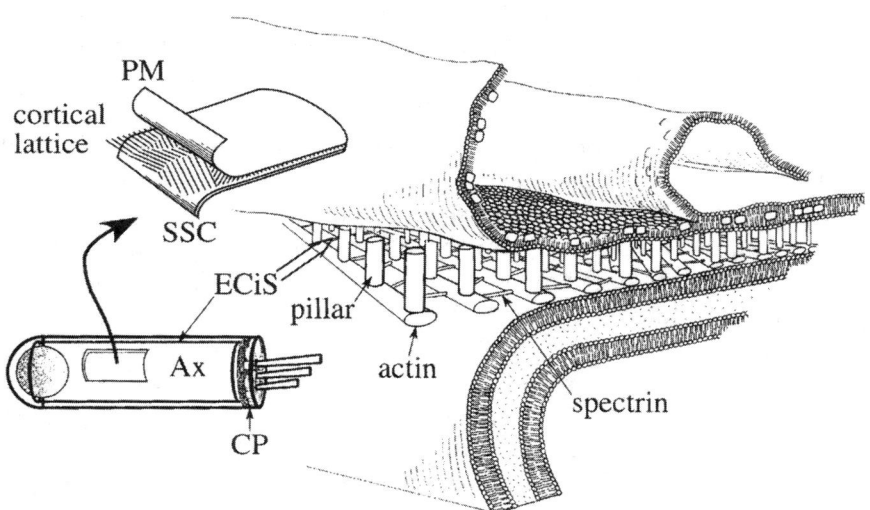

Figure 2–2. Diagram of outer hair cell showing organization of lateral wall components. Axial core (Ax), extracisternal space (ECiS), subsurface cisterna (SSC), cuticular plate (CP), plasma membrane (PM). From Brownell and Papel (1998).

wall is ~100 nm (about 25% the wavelength of visible light and an order of magnitude less than the thickness of the OHC's trilaminate apical pole). The plasma membrane (PM) is again the outermost layer. The membrane-bound subsurface cisterna (SSC) forms the innermost layer. The membranes of the SSC are continuous with those of the canalicular reticulum. Sandwiched between the PM and the SSC is a cytoskeletal matrix called the cortical lattice (CL). The CL is composed of cytoskeletal proteins, two of which (F-actin and spectrin) are found in the cuticular plate.

The Lateral Wall Plasma Membrane

The composition of the lateral wall plasma membrane differs from that of the apical pole plasma membrane. Mechanoelectrical transduction channels and purinergic receptor channels are located only in the apical pole plasma membrane (Brownell et al., 2001). A tight junction complex is found at the boundary between the apical and lateral wall plasma membrane domains and prevents diffusion of integral membrane proteins between the two. The lipid composition of OHC membranes is unknown. Fluorescent labeling studies suggest that lateral wall membranes contain less cholesterol than the apical and basal plasma membrane (Nguyen & Brownell 1998) and that the plasma membrane does not retain cholesterol (Oghalai, Tran, Raphael, Nakagawa, & Brownell, 1999). The lipid composition of the membrane can modulate the activity of membrane proteins. Just as low membrane cholesterol is required for rhodopsin to undergo a conformational change in response to light (Boesze-Battaglia & Albert, 1990) it may be that low cholesterol is required for OHC electromotility. Immunohistochemical studies reveal that lateral wall membranes contain a modified anion exchanger AE2 (Kalinec, Kalinec, Negrini, & Kachar, 1997), a water channel protein (Belyantseva, Frolenkov, Wade, Mammano, & Kachar, 2000), a sugar transporter (Belyantseva, Adler, Curi, Frolenkov, & Kachar, 2000; Geleoc, Casalotti, Forge, & Ashmore, 1999; Nakazawa, Spicer, & Schulte, 1995), and a protein involved in OHC electromotilty called prestin (Belyantseva, Adler, et al., 2000; Zheng et al., 2000). There is also functional evidence for differences in integral membrane proteins between the lateral wall plasma membrane and the OHC basal pole even though there is no obvious diffusion barrier between these membranes. For instance, there appear to be little or no voltage-gated ion channels along the lateral wall, which are concentrated instead at the base of the cell (Santos-Sacchi, Huang,

& Wu, 1997) along with ACh receptor channels (Blanchet, Erostegui, Sugasawa, & Dulan, 1996). The integral membrane proteins that are unique to either may partition differently based on the lipid composition of the different domains and/or differences in membrane curvature (Ramaswamy, Toner, & Prost, 2000). It is also possible that the integral membrane proteins are evenly distributed in the two domains but their functional expression is altered by either the lipid composition (Boesze-Battaglia & Albert, 1990) or membrane curvature (Hubner et al., 1998).

The Lateral Wall Subsurface Cisterna

The molecular composition of the SSC is unknown. Its phospholipid composition, complement of integral membrane proteins, and the content of the narrow (~20 nm) lumen between the inner and outer SSC membranes remain to be identified. The SSC structurally resembles the endoplasmic reticulum (ER), is stained with both ER and Golgi body markers (Pollice & Brownell, 1993), but shows no evidence of belonging to the PM-ER-Golgi membrane pool (Siegel & Brownell, 1986). Dyes that stain the SSC also stain the canalicular reticulum (Brownell & Oghalai, 2000; Oghalai et al., 1998; Pollice & Brownell, 1993) and confirm ultrastructural studies that show continuity between the membranes of the canalicular reticulum and the SSC (Spicer et al., 1998). These studies show continuity between the membranes of the SSC and the outer membrane of mitochondria, consistent with the fact that lipid dyes for mitochondria will also stain the SSC (Forge, Zajic, Li, Nevill, & Schacht, 1993; Pollice & Brownell, 1993). The low cholesterol of lateral wall membranes is consistent with the absence of cholesterol in mitochondrial membranes (Yeagle, 1993). Most of the cell's mitochondria are found just medial to the SSC.

While the function of the SSC is unknown, it partitions the cytoplasm into two domains, the axial core and the ~30-nm wide extracisternal space (ECiS). The axial core is the larger of the two compartments. It is central to the SSC and extends from the cell nucleus in the base to the canalicular reticulum in the apex. The very center of the axial core is typically devoid of filamentous cytoskeletal proteins and other subcellular organelles (Raphael, Athey, Wang, Lee, & Altschuler, 1994). The ECiS, in contrast, represents a very small portion of the OHC's volume, yet it is where the filamentous proteins that maintain the OHC's cylindrical shape are located. The SSC may function to provide a small reaction volume for the enzymes that control cytoskeletal protein (Forge et al., 1993; Kakehata et al., 2000).

The Lateral Wall Cortical Lattice

The CL is the matrix of preferentially oriented cytoskeletal proteins located in the ECiS and is mechanically anisotropic. This layer of the lateral wall appears to be a continuation of the cuticular plate. The OHC cuticular plate is larger than the cuticular plate of other hair cells. It spans the width of the cell and joins the CL at the lateral wall plasma membrane immediately below the apical tight junctions. It is thicker than the cuticular plates of other hair cells, and stereocilia rootlets do not penetrate it (Liberman 1987; Takasaka, Shinkawa, Hashimoto, Watanuki, & Kawamoto, 1983). The thickness of the OHC cuticular plate increases as it gets closer to the lateral wall so that it is concave apically. The cuticular plate in all other hair cells is convex; they are thickest in the center and do not reach the lateral membranes. The cuticular plate of most hair cells appears to be a random array of filamentous cytoskeletal proteins. In the OHC, cuticular plate spectrin is organized in bundles that radiate toward the lateral wall away from the F-actin-based stereocilia rootlets (Raphael et al., 1994). The orthogonal orientation of spectrin and rootlet F-actin may be a unique feature of the OHC cuticular plate.

The perpendicular arrangement of spectrin and F-actin in the OHC cuticular plate continues in the orthotopic organization of the CL (see Figure 2–3). Filaments of F-actin are spaced ~40 nm apart and cross-linked with molecules of spectrin. The CL extends the length of the lateral wall and is organized in microdomains defined by regions of parallel actin filaments. The orientation of the actin differs between the microdomains but on average is circumferential (Holley, Kalinec, & Kachar, 1992). The mean orientation of the spectrin is longitudinal. Radially oriented pillars of unknown composition tether the plasma membrane to the parallel bands of F-actin that lie adjacent to the SSC. The circumferential bands of F-actin in the CL provide the tensile force that maintains the OHC's cylindrical shape against its elevated cytoplasmic turgor pressure (Brownell, 1990). The same studies that show F-actin in the CL also reveal a conspicuous absence in the OHC axial core (Brownell & Oghalai, 2000; Oghalai et al., 1998; Raphael et al., 1994). The poor expression of long chain cytoskeletal elements in the OHC axial core permits hydraulic force transmission to the ends of the cell without dissipating energy through the deformation of a viscoelastic cytoskeleton (Brownell, 1990; Brownell & Popel, 1998; Brownell et al., 2001). In addition to the circumferential F-actin in the CL, bundles of F-actin contribute to the mechanical rigidity of stereocilia and anchor them in the cuticular plate. The length, width, and spatial orientation of each stereocilium is determined by its bundle. Clearly, F-actin is important for the structural organization of both the OHC CL and its apical pole.

Because OHCs are terminally differentiated cells and required for normal mammalian hearing, they must survive the life span of the animal. The longevity of the cells requires that their cellular components (such as the CL and cuticular plate) recycle. The initial expression and homeostatic regulation of structures as precisely ordered as the CL and cuticular plate present a unique challenge for the cell-signaling pathways that regulate cytoskeletal protein polymerization. The regulation of many cytoskeletal proteins is under the control of the small GTPase pathways that involve RAC, RHO, and CDC42. Kalinec, Zhang, Urrutia, and Kalinec (2000) have recently shown these enzymes are particularly well represented in the cuticular plate and CL of the OHC. By blocking different portions of the small GTPase pathways that regulate cytoskeleton polymerization, the magnitude of the electromotile response in the presence of ACh (Dallos et al., 1997; Kalinec et al., 2000; Sziklai, He, & Dallos, 1996) can either be increased or decreased. Focal, free radical damage to the lateral wall damages the cortical lattice, and the cell undergoes circumferential ballooning at the level of the lesion followed by a return to its original shape. The magnitude of the cell's response and the time course of its recovery from the damage can be modulated by agents associated with the regulation of cytoskeletal polymerization (Zhao, Shellenberger, Shope, & Brownell, 2001). The demonstrated turnover and self-repair of the OHC lateral wall cytoskeleton has implications for the control of OHC mechanics. Because ACh can modulate the signal transduction pathways, these results suggest that the efferent olivocochlear bundle regulation of cochlear function may involve a change in CL mechanics. A restricted volume like that of the ECiS would enhance the effect of the small GTPases on the CL because the cytosolic GTPases are translocated to membranes on activation (Kakehata et al., 2000). A location close to the membranes reduces the response time. It remains to be determined if the time course is consistent with that observed for olivocochlear bundle stimulation effects on cochlear transduction.

The orthotopic relation between F-actin and spectrin in both the cuticular plate and the CL is another feature whose origin requires an explanation. Cell signaling pathways somehow result in the radial orientation of spectrin in the cuticular plate and the longitudinal orientation of spectrin in the CL. The mechanism restricting F-actin polymerization in the circumferential direction in the CL is not obvious. The longitudinal orientation of stereocilia F-actin may result from the restriction of its polymerization/depolymerization by the PM. It is has been proposed that the OHC lateral wall PM is organized in longitudinal ripples (Oghalai, Zhao, Kutz, & Brownell, 2000; Raphael, Popel, & Brownell, 2000). Longitudinal PM ripples may contribute to F-actin orientation in the CL. In both cases the F-actin orientation is at right angles to the resultant force vector associated with the two subcellular domains.

MECHANICAL FORCE GENERATION BY HAIR CELLS

Hair cells generate active mechanical force using motor mechanisms associated either with their stereocilia and/or their lateral wall. Stereocilia generate force at right angles to the hair cell's longitudinal axis, parallel to the bundle's axis of symmetry. The lateral wall generates force parallel to the outer hair cell axis. In both cases the mechanism is not known. The bundle motor unit is associated with mechano-electrical transduction channels, and the bundle's net force is directly proportional to the number of stereocilia. The characteristics of the OHC electromotility (Brownell, 1990; Brownell & Popel, 1998; Brownell et al., 2001) may be compared with the emerging characteristics of the bundle mechanism. The motor mechanism underlying OHC electromotility generates forces with gains of ~50 pN/mV at frequencies approaching 100 kHz (Brownell et al., 2001; Frank, Hemmert, & Gummer, 1999). Two plausible molecular mechanisms for OHC electromotility have been proposed based on an electromechanical transduction process in the PM. One is driven by in-plane conformational changes of a motor protein (Dallos, Hallworth, & Evans, 1993; Huang & Santos-Sacchi, 1994; Iwasa, 1994; Iwasa & Adachi, 1997; Iwasa & Chadwick, 1993; Kalinec, Holley, Iwasa, Lim, & Kachar, 1992) and the other by out-of-plane flexoelectric bending (Raphael et al., 2000). The motor protein is thought to possess an associated charge density that varies between 5,000 to 50,000 elements/μm^2 depending on the length of the cell (Santos-Sacchi, Kakehata, Kikuchi, Katori, & Takasaka, 1998), or ~15–30 million elements per cell. In the membrane-bending flexoelectric model the motor unit is a longitudinally oriented ripple with a width of ~40 nm or ~25,000 per mm. A 50 mm long cell will have > 1 million motor units. The number of mechanoelectrical transduction channels determines the number of bundle motor units so that the bundle's net force is proportional to the number of stereocilia (≤ 300). The number of motor units in the lateral wall is between 10^3 to 10^4 times the number of bundle motor units. The increased number of lateral wall motor units makes the relatively large OHC electromotility force production possible. A cochlear amplifier based on stereocilia appears to have reached a limit at around 10 kHz. Increasing the frequency range for hearing another order of magnitude requires the negative damping force of the cochlear amplifier to increase by the same amount. The surface area at the apical pole cannot sustain 10^4 stereocilia. The structural and functional features of the apical pole formed the basis for a force transduction mechanism based on the direct conversion of membrane potential to mechanical force. It is intriguing that a recent study of turtle hair cell bundle force transduction describes a possible voltage-dependent process in addition to the fast and slow calcium-dependent mechanisms (Ricci et al., 2000).

FUNCTIONAL CHARACTERISTICS OF BACTERIAL TYPE-A GLIDING

Many bacteria colonies appear to "glide" along surfaces using a form of locomotion called gliding (Burchard, 1981; McBride, 2000; Pate, 1988). These primitive prokaryotes lack flagella or other obvious motility organelles. The molecular basis of the locomotor mechanism (like OHC electromotility) is enigmatic, and a variety of models have been proposed (Burchard, 1981). Many gliding bacteria are rod shaped, having diameters of about 500 nm and lengths < 1,000 nm (wider and shorter than most stereocilia). When observed under a microscope individual gliding bacteria display either type-S and/or type-A locomotion.

Type-S or "social" motility typically involves at least two bacteria that execute twitching movements (Kaiser, 1979). This form of gliding motility is thought to involve the extension of a thin extracellular filament or pilus by one bacterium that attaches to another bacterium. The filament is then retracted bringing the two bacteria together. The pilus is extended from one end of the bacterium reminiscent of stereocilia tip links. The retraction force has been measured and can reach values of ~80 pN (Merz, So, & Sheetz, 2000).

Type-A or "adventurous" gliding motility describes the movement of a single bacterium across a surface. The cell moves parallel to its long axis at speeds that can reach 50 mm/sec (Hoiczyk, 2000). The cell's longitudinal movement is often accompanied by species-specific revolutions around the cells long axis (Burchard, 1981; Hoiczyk & Baumeister, 1995). There is no apparent bending, rippling, or change in cell length under the light microscope. Microbeads attached to a gliding bacterium move along the cell surface parallel to the cell's long axis (Lapidus & Berg, 1982) at speeds comparable to their locomotion. Membrane potential rather than ATP drives type-A gliding motility (Pate, 1988), like OHC electromotility. Lanthanides block gliding motility (Pitta, Sherwood, Kobel, & Berg, 1997) and OHC electromotility (Kakehata & Santos-Sacchi, 1996). OHCs and gliding bacteria share a surprising number of structural motifs.

STRUCTURAL FEATURES OF TYPE-A GLIDING BACTERIA

Bacteria, like OHCs, are cellular hydrostats. A hydrostat is a mechanical structure formed from an elastic outer shell enclosing a pressurized core. The outer hair cell is normally pressurized (or turgid), and electromotility diminishes and vanishes if the cell becomes flaccid (Shehata, Brownell, & Dieler, 1991). While plant and bacterial cells have pressurized fluid cores, the OHC is the only vertebrate cell known to share this feature. Bacteria, like all prokaryotes, do not have the cytoskeletal proteins of eukaryotes. The poorly developed central cytoskeleton of OHCs is therefore another similarity. The elastic outer wall of both the OHC and bacteria is made of three layers (Figure 2–3). The most peripheral membrane in the bacterial cell wall is called the outer membrane and it establishes a permeability barrier in which transport molecules are located. Its innermost membrane is called the cytoplasmic membrane. The cytoplasmic membrane contains proton pumps and other integral membrane proteins crucial to the bacterial energy utilization. In between the membranes is found the peptidoglycan layer serving a cytoskeletal function similar to that of the OHC's cortical lattice. Cholesterol is found only in eukaryotic membranes. The low concentration of cholesterol in mitochondrial membranes reflects their prokaryotic origins. The low concentration of cholesterol in the OHC PM and SSC (Forge, 1991; Nguyen & Brownell, 1998) is yet another similarity between the OHC lateral wall and the bacterial cell wall. These similarities may contribute to the fact that both OHCs and gram-negative bacteria are particularly vulnerable to aminoglycosides.

Transmission electronmicroscopy reveals that the outer membrane of type-A gliding bacteria is rippled (Figure 2–3) much like the plasma membrane of the OHC (Adams, Ashworth, & Nelmes, 1999; Dickson,

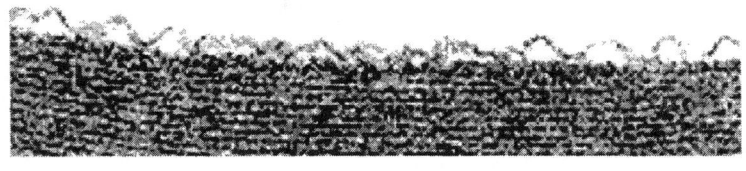

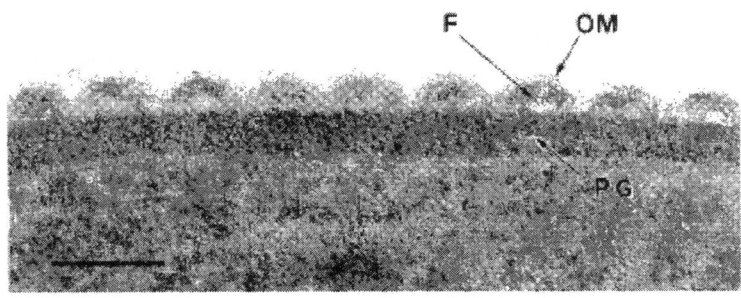

Figure 2–3. Electronmicrographs of the OHC lateral wall (top) and the cell wall of a type-A gliding bacteria. OHC image from Dieler et al. (1991) 21; bottom image from Adams et al. (1999).

Kouprach, Humphrey, & Marshall, 1980). When the cells are prepared using rapid freezing techniques the outer membrane appears flat, and paracrystalline arrays of particles are observed (Hoiczyk & Baumeister, 1995). The OHC plasma membrane also appears flat and contains a paracrystalline array of large particles when subjected to the same treatment (Gulley & Reese, 1977; Kalinec et al., 1992). The ripples of type-A gliding bacteria spiral around the cell, and the direction of the spiral is in the same direction as the rotation of the cell as it glides (Halfen & Castenholz, 1970; Hoiczyk & Baumeister, 1995). The association between the orientation of the ripples and the rotation has led to the proposal of a screw mechanism for the gliding, in which small surface waves travel longitudinally (or helically) along the surface of the cell and pull the cell along the surface (Halfen & Castenholz, 1970). A variation of this model has been proposed to explain the ability of a cyanobacteria species to swim in the absence of flagella (Ehlers, Samuel, Berg, & Montgomery, 1996; Stone & Samuel, 1996). These models require traveling waves with an amplitude of ~20 nm to account for the swimming. The magnitude of the traveling wave is the same order of magnitude as the OHC PM ripple height change required for electromotile length changes. OHC length changes have been postulated to result from nanoscale changes in PM ripples (Figure 2–4). The magnitude of the OHC PM ripple height change is based on the geometry of the PM and cortical lattice attachments

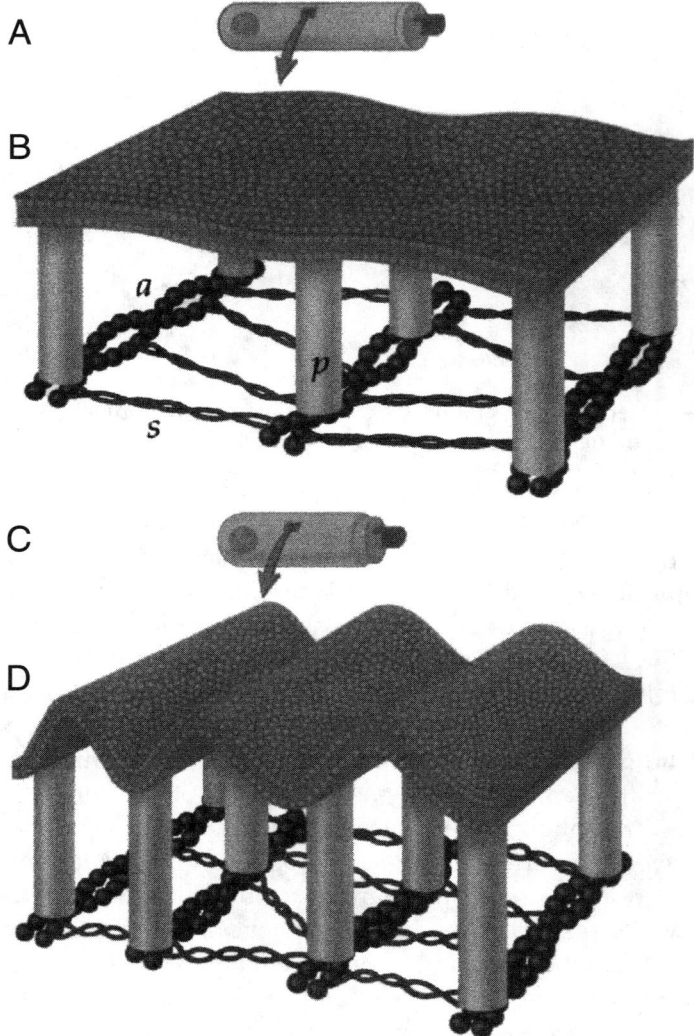

Figure 2–4. Postulated nanoscale membrane rippling within the lateral wall of the OHC. Pillars (*p*); actin filaments (*a*); spectrin (*s*). (A & C) The OHC when hyperpolarized and depolarized, respectively. (B & D) Alterations in membrane curvature associated with electromotile length changes. From Oghalai et al. (1999).

(Oghalai et al., 2000; Raphael et al., 2000). The OHC length changes result from the simultaneous activation of all the motor elements in the lateral wall. This differs from the bacterial gliding and swimming waves that travel longitudinally.

The protein prestin is involved in OHC electromotility and shows homologies to sulfate transporters (Zheng et al., 2000). Sulfate transporters are members of an ancient family of integral membrane proteins that facilitate diffusion across membranes. Sulfate-reducing bacteria utilize sulfate transporters as they help to purify the environment. Diffusion-facilitating transporters do not utilize ATP directly, and neither their precise structure nor the way they work in the membrane is understood. They are typically imagined as opening to one or the other side of the membrane then closing on that side while opening on the other. The process resembles a pressure lock on a submarine, and selected substances are moved across the membrane. Substances that fail to match the selectivity of the opening are not transported. It is useful to consider the implications of placing such a transport mechanism in a curved membrane. Membrane curvature establishes a differential tension between the inner and outer membrane leaflets. Transporter opening and closing would be in response to tension changes in the leaflet. The degree of membrane curvature would determine which face of the transporter is open, and a change in curvature would activate transport. Coupling local membrane curvature to the cell's transmembrane potential may help to explain why voltage-gated ion channels capable of supporting action potentials are found in many prokaryotes.

THE HAIR CELL BASAL POLE: ELECTROCHEMICAL TRANSDUCTION

The basal end of hair cells is specialized for synaptic communication with afferent and efferent fibers in the VIIIth nerve. The synapses at afferent fiber terminals modulate the firing of the postsynaptic fibers based on the magnitude and temporal properties of hair cell receptor potentials. Presynaptic structures found in hair cells are similar to those found in retinal photoreceptors (Brownell, 1982; Siegel & Brownell, 1981). These synapses are believed responsible for the high rates of both spontaneous and driven firing rates of auditory/vestibular neurons and, in the case of auditory nerve fibers, permit phase locking at frequencies > 5 kHz (Koppl, 1997). The ability to initiate action potential at a given phase of a stimulus sinusoid calls for precise temporal control of the neurotransmitter. The precise temporal synchronization with the hair cell receptor potential occurs at intensities below that defined as threshold, where the discharge rate is greater than the spontaneous firing rate. The temporal precision is even more remarkable because the preferred phase angle is invariant with intensity at best frequency. The molecular mechanisms responsible for the temporal precision have yet to be identified. The curvature of vesicle membranes is close to the limit that lipid double layers can achieve without being pulled apart by surface tension. The plasma membrane ripples in the outer cell lateral wall and the outer membrane ripples in the bacterial cell wall approach the curvature of synaptic vesicles. Vesicular fusion is a mechanical event, and over the past decade many of the molecules that control the docking of the vesicle with the presynaptic membrane have been discovered. Some of these are thought to act by matching the difference in surface tension between the highly curved vesicle and the relatively flat presynaptic membrane. Once fusion occurs neurotransmitter release is determined by mechanics. The membrane mechanics may in turn be subject to flexoelectric forces that convert the receptor potentials to mechanical force and "squirt" the neurotransmitter into the synaptic cleft. Electromechanical control of membrane curvature offers a mechanism that may contribute to neurotransmitter kinetics.

The evolutionary pressure for increasing the upper frequency limits of hearing appears to have lead to the membrane-based electromechanical force transduction found in the OHC lateral wall. The structural and functional features of the apical end of hair cells have extended to the lateral wall. It is also possible that the exocytotic mechanisms at the basal end of hair cells, like the calcium-based adaptation motors at the apical end, reached a frequency limit and are augmented by an electromechanical force transduction similar to that found in the lateral wall. It remains to be determined whether the requirement for auditory frequency processing by hair cells uses mechanisms similar to those of bacterial motility that date back to the origin of life on earth.

Acknowledgments: I would like to thank Drs. R. A. Eatock, J. Oghalai, A. S. Popel, R. M. Raphael, and F. Sachs for helpful discussion and comments. This work was supported by National Institutes of Health grants DC02775 and DC00354.

REFERENCES

Adams, D. G., Ashworth, D, & Nelmes B. (1999). Fibrillar array in the cell wall of a gliding filamentous cyanobacterium. *Journal of Bacteriology, 181*(3), 884–892.

Allman, J. (1999). *Evolving brains.* New York: Scientific American Library.

Belyantseva, I. A., Adler, H. J., Curi, R., Frolenkov, G. I., & Kachar, B. (2000a). Expression and localization of prestin and the sugar transporter GLUT-5 during development of electromotility in cochlear outer hair cells. *Journal of Neuroscience, 20*(24), RC116.

Belyantseva, I. A., Frolenkov, G. I., Wade, J. B., Mammano, F., & Kachar, B. (2000b). Water permeability of cochlear outer hair cells: Characterization and relationship to electromotility. *Journal of Neuroscience, 20*(24), 8996–9003.

Blanchet, C., Erostegui, C., Sugasawa, M., & Dulon, D. (1996). Acetylcholine-induced potassium current of guinea pig outer hair cells: Its dependence on a calcium influx through nicotinic-like receptors. *Journal of Neuroscience, 16*(8), 2574–2584.

Boesze-Battaglia, K., & Albert, A. D. (1990). Cholesterol modulation of photoreceptor function in bovine retinal rod outer segments. *Journal of Biological Chemistry, 265*(34), 20727–20730.

Brownell, W. E. (1982). Cochlear transduction: An integrative model and review. *Hearing Research, 6,* 335–360.

Brownell, W. E. (1990). Outer hair cell electromotility and otoacoustic emissions. *Ear and Hearing, 11*(2), 82–92.

Brownell, W. E., & Oghalai, J. S. (2000). Structural basis of outer hair cell motility or where's the motor? In D. Lim (Ed.), *Cell and molecular biology of the ear* (pp. 69–83). New York: Academic/Plenum Press.

Brownell, W. E., & Popel, A. S. (1998). Electrical and mechanical anatomy of the outer hair cell. In A. R. Palmer, A. Rees, A. Q. Summerfield, & R. Meddis (Eds.), *Psychophysical and physiological advances in hearing* (pp. 89–96). London: Whurr.

Brownell, W. E., Spector, A. A., Raphael, R. M., & Popel, A. S. (2001). Micro- and nanomechanics of the cochlear outer hair cell. *Annual Review of Biomedical Engineering, 3,* 169–194.

Burchard, R. P. (1981). Gliding motility of prokaryotes: Ultrastructure, physiology, and genetics. *Annual Review of Microbiology, 35,* 497–529.

Choe, Y., Magnasco, M. O., & Hudspeth, A. J. (1998). A model for amplification of hair-bundle motion by cyclical binding of Ca2+ to mechanoelectrical-transduction channels. *Proceedings of the National Academy of Sciences, USA, 95*(26), 15321–15326.

Corey, D. P., & Hudspeth, A. J. (1979). Response latency of vertebrate hair cells. *Biophysical Journal, 26*(3), 499–506.

Crawford, A. C., & Fettiplace, R. (1985). The mechanical properties of ciliary bundles of turtle cochlear hair cells. *Journal of Physiology (London), 364,* 359–379.

Dallos, P., Hallworth, R., & Evans, B. N. (1993). Theory of electrically driven shape changes of cochlear outer hair cells. *Journal of Neurophysiology, 70*(1), 299–323.

Dallos, P., He, D. Z., Lin, X., Sziklai, I., Mehta, S., & Evans, B. N. (1997). Acetylcholine, outer hair cell electromotility, and the cochlear amplifier. *Journal of Neuroscience, 17*(6), 2212–2226.

Davis, H. (1983). An active process in cochlear mechanics. *Hearing Research, 9*(1), 79–90.

Denk, W., & Webb, W. W. (1992). Forward and reverse transduction at the limit of sensitivity studied by correlating electrical and mechanical fluctuations in frog saccular hair cells. *Hearing Research, 60*(1), 89–102.

Dickson, M. R., Kouprach, S., Humphrey, B. A., & Marshall, K. C. (1980). Does gliding motility depend on undulating membranes? *Micron, 11*, 381–382.

Dieler, R., Shehata-Dieler, W. E., & Brownell, W. E. (1991). Concomitant salicylate-induced alterations of outer hair cell subsurface cisternae and electromotility. *Journal of Neurocytology, 20*(8), 637–653.

Eatock, R. A. (2000). Adaptation in hair cells. *Annual Review of Neuroscience, 23*, 285–314.

Ehlers, K. M., Samuel, A. D., Berg, H. C., & Montgomery, R. (1996). Do cyanobacteria swim using traveling surface waves? *Proceedings of the National Academy of Sciences, USA, 93*(16), 8340–8343.

Forge, A. (1991). Structural features of the lateral walls in mammalian cochlear outer hair cells. *Cell and Tissue Research, 265*(3), 473–483.

Forge, A., Zajic, G., Li, L., Nevill, G., & Schacht, J. (1993). Structural variability of the sub-surface cisternae in intact, isolated outer hair cells shown by fluorescent labelling of intracellular membranes and freeze-fracture. *Hearing Research, 64*(2), 175–183.

Frank, G., Hemmert, W., & Gummer, A. W. (1999). Limiting dynamics of high-frequency electromechanical transduction of outer hair cells. *Proceedings of the National Academy of Sciences, USA, 96*(8), 4420–4425.

Geleoc, G. S., Casalotti, S. O., Forge, A., & Ashmore, J. F. (1999). A sugar transporter as a candidate for the outer hair cell motor. *Nature Neuroscience, 2*(8), 713–719.

Gold, T. (1948). Hearing. II. The physical basis of the action of the cochlea. *Proceedings of the Royal Society of London, Series B, Biological Sciences, 135*, 492–498.

Gulley, R. L., & Reese, T. S. (1977). Regional specialization of the hair cell plasmalemma in the organ of Corti. *Anatomical Record, 189*(1), 109–123.

Halfen, L. N., & Castenholz, R. W. (1970). Gliding in a blue-green alga: A possible mechanism. *Nature, 225*(238), 1163–1165.

Hoiczyk, E. (2000). Gliding motility in cyanobacterial: Observations and possible explanations. *Archives of Microbiology, 174*(1-2), 11–17.

Hoiczyk, E., & Baumeister, W. (1995). Envelope structure of four gliding filamentous cyanobacteria. *Journal of Bacteriology, 177*(9), 2387–2395.

Holley, M. C., Kalinec, F., & Kachar, B. (1992). Structure of the cortical cytoskeleton in mammalian outer hair cells. *Journal of Cell Science, 102*(Pt 3), 569–580.

Howard, J., & Hudspeth, A. J. (1987). Mechanical relaxation of the hair bundle mediates adaptation in mechanoelectrical transduction by the bullfrog's saccular hair cell. *Proceedings of the National Academy of Sciences, USA, 84*(9), 3064–3068.

Huang, G., Santos-Sacchi, J. (1994). Motility voltage sensor of the outer hair cell resides within the lateral plasma membrane. *Proceedings of the National Academy of Sciences, USA, 91*(25), 12268–12272.

Hubner, S., Couvillon, A. D., Kas, J. A., Bankaitis, V. A., Vegners, R., Carpenter, C. L., & Janmey, P. A. (1998). Enhancement of phosphoinositide 3-kinase (PI 3-kinase) activity by membrane curvature and inositol-phospholipid-binding peptides. *European Journal of Biochemistry, 258*(2), 846–853.

Hudspeth, A. J. (1997). Mechanical amplification of stimuli by hair cells. *Current Opinion in Neurobiology, 7*(4), 480–486.

Iwasa, K. H. (1994). A membrane motor model for the fast motility of the outer hair cell. *The Journal of the Acoustical Society of America, 96*(4), 2216–2224.

Iwasa, K. H., & Adachi, M. (1997). Force generation in the outer hair cell of the cochlea. *Biophysical Journal, 73*(1), 546–555.

Iwasa, K. H, & Chadwick, R. S. (1993). Factors influencing the length change of an auditory outer hair cell in a tight-fitting capillary [letter]. *The Journal of the Acoustical Society of America, 94*(2 Pt 1), 1156–1159.

Kachar, B., Parakkal, M., Kurc, M., Zhao, Y., & Gillespie, P. G. (2000). High-resolution structure of hair-cell tip links [In Process Citation]. *Proceedings of the National Academy of Sciences, USA, 97*(24), 13336–13341.

Kaiser, D. (1979). Social gliding is correlated with the presence of pili in Myxococcus xanthus. *Proceedings of the National Academy of Sciences, USA, 76*(11), 5952–5956.

Kakehata, S., Dallos, P., Brownell, W. E., Iwasa, K. H., Kachar, B., Kalinec, F., Ikeda, K., & Takasaka, T. (2000). Current concept of outer hair cell motility. *Auris Nasus Larynx, 27*(4), 349–355.

Kakehata, S., & Santos-Sacchi, J. (1996). Effects of salicylate and lanthanides on outer hair cell motility and associated gating charge. *Journal of Neuroscience, 16*(16), 4881–4889.

Kalinec, F., Holley, M. C., Iwasa, K. H., Lim, D. J., & Kachar, B. (1992). A membrane-based force generation mechanism in auditory sensory cells. *Proceedings of the National Academy of Sciences, USA, 89*(18), 8671–8675.

Kalinec, F., Kalinec, G., Negrini, C., & Kachar, B. (1997). Immunolocalization of anion exchanger 2alpha in auditory sensory hair cells. *Hearing Research, 110*(1-2), 141–146.

Kalinec, F., Zhang, M., Urrutia, R., & Kalinec, G. (2000). Rho GTPases mediate the regulation of cochlear outer hair cell motility by acetylcholine. *The Journal of Biological Chemistry, 275*(36), 28000–28005.

Koppl, C. (1997). Phase locking to high frequencies in the auditory nerve and cochlear nucleus magnocellularis of the barn owl, *Tyto alba*. *Journal of Neuroscience, 17*(9), 3312–3321.

Lapidus, I. R., & Berg, H. C. (1982). Gliding motility of Cytophaga sp. strain U67. *Journal of Bacteriology, 151*(1), 384–398.

Liberman, M. C. (1987). Chronic ultrastructural changes in acoustic trauma: Serial-section reconstruction of stereocilia and cuticular plates. *Hearing Research, 26*(1), 65–88.

Manley, G. A. (2000). Cochlear mechanisms from a phylogenetic viewpoint. *Proceedings of the National Academy of Sciences, USA, 97*(22), 11736–11743.

Martin, P., & Hudspeth, A. J. (1999). Active hair-bundle movements can amplify a hair cell's response to oscillatory mechanical stimuli. *Proceedings of the National Academy of Sciences, USA, 96*(25), 14306–14311.

McBride, M. J. (2000). Bacterial gliding motility: Mechanisms and mysteries. *ASM News, 66*, 203–210.

Merz, A. J., So, M., & Sheetz, M. P. (2000). Pilus retraction powers bacterial twitching motility. *Nature, 407*(6800), 98–102.

Nakazawa, K., Spicer, S. S., & Schulte, B. A. (1995). Postnatal expression of the facilitated glucose transporter, GLUT 5, in gerbil outer hair cells. *Hearing Research, 82*(1), 93–99.

Nguyen, T. V., & Brownell, W. E. (1998). Contribution of membrane cholesterol to outer hair cell lateral wall stiffness. *Otolaryngology and Head and Neck Surgery, 119*(1), 14–20.

Oghalai, J. S., Patel, A. A., Nakagawa, T., & Brownell, W. E. (1998). Fluorescence-imaged microdeformation of the outer hair cell lateral wall. *Journal of Neuroscience, 18*(1), 48–58.

Oghalai, J. S., Tran, T. D., Raphael, R. M., Nakagawa, T., & Brownell, W. E. (1999). Transverse and lateral mobility in outer hair cell lateral wall membranes. *Hearing Research, 135*(1-2), 19–28.

Oghalai, J. S, Zhao, H. B., Kutz, J. W., & Brownell, W. E. (2000). Voltage- and tension-dependent lipid mobility in the outer hair cell plasma membrane. *Science, 287*(5453), 658–661.

Osborne, M. P, Comis, S. D., & Pickles, J. O. (1984). Morphology and cross-linkage of stereocilia in the guinea-pig labyrinth examined without the use of osmium as a fixative. *Cell and Tissue Research, 237*(1), 43–48.

Pate, J. L. (1988). Gliding motility in procaryotic cells. *Canadian Journal of Microbiology, 34*, 459–465.

Pickles, J. O., Comis, S. D., & Osborne, M. P. (1984). Cross-links between stereocilia in the guinea pig organ of Corti, and their possible relation to sensory transduction. *Hearing Research, 15*(2), 103–112.

Pitta, T. P., Sherwood, E. E., Kobel, A. M., & Berg, H. C. (1997). Calcium is required for swimming by the nonflagellated cyanobacterium Synechococcus strain WH8113. *Journal of Bacteriology, 179*(8), 2524–2528.

Pollice, P. A., & Brownell, W. E. (1993). Characterization of the outer hair cell's lateral wall membranes. *Hearing Research, 70*(2), 187–196.

Ramaswamy, S., Toner, J., & Prost, J. (2000). Nonequilibrium fluctuations, traveling waves, and instabilities in active membranes. *Physical Review Letters, 84*(15), 3494–3497.

Raphael, R. M., Popel, A. S., & Brownell, W. E. (2000). A membrane bending model of outer hair cell electromotility. *Biophysical Journal, 78*(6), 2844–2862.

Raphael, Y., Athey, B. D., Wang, Y., Lee, M. K., & Altschuler, R. A. (1994). F-actin, tubulin and spectrin in the organ of Corti: Comparative distribution in different cell types and mammalian species. *Hearing Research, 76*(1-2), 173–187.

Ricci, A. J., Crawford, A. C., & Fettiplace, R. (2000). Active hair bundle motion linked to fast transducer adaptation in auditory hair cells. *Journal of Neuroscience, 20*(19), 7131–7142.

Rusch, A., & Thurm, U. (1990). Spontaneous and electrically induced movements of ampullary kinocilia and stereovilli. *Hearing Research, 48*(3), 247–263.

Santos-Sacchi, J., Huang, G. J., & Wu, M. (1997). Mapping the distribution of outer hair cell voltage-dependent conductances by electrical amputation. *Biophysical Journal, 73*(3), 1424–1429.

Santos-Sacchi, J., Kakehata, S., Kikuchi, T., Katori, Y., & Takasaka, T. (1998). Density of motility-related charge in the outer hair cell of the guinea pig is inversely related to best frequency. *Neuroscience Letters, 256*(3), 155–158.

Shehata, W. E., Brownell, W. E., & Dieler, R. (1991). Effects of salicylate on shape, electromotility and membrane characteristics of isolated outer hair cells from guinea pig cochlea. *Acta Oto-laryngologica (Stockh), 111*(4), 707–718.

Siegel, J. H., & Brownell, W. E. (1981). Presynaptic bodies in outer hair cells of the chinchilla organ of Corti. *Brain Research, 220,* 188–193.

Siegel, J. H., & Brownell, W. E. (1986). Synaptic and golgi membrane recycling in cochlear hair cells. *Journal of Neurocytology, 15,* 311–328.

Spicer, S. S., Thomopoulos, G. N., & Schulte, B. A. (1998). Cytologic evidence for mechanisms of K+ transport and genesis of Hensen bodies and subsurface cisternae in outer hair cells. *The Anatomical Record, 251*(1), 97–113.

Stone, H. A., & Samuel, A. D. (1996). Propulsion of Microorganisms by Surface Distortions. *Physical Review Letters, 77*(19), 4102–4104.

Sziklai, I., He, D. Z., & Dallos, P. (1996). Effect of acetylcholine and GABA on the transfer function of electromotility in isolated outer hair cells. *Hearing Research, 95*(1-2), 87–99.

Takasaka, T., Shinkawa, H., Hashimoto, S., Watanuki, K., & Kawamoto, K. (1983). High-voltage electron microscopic study of the inner ear. Technique and preliminary results. *The Annals of Otology, Rhinology, and Laryngology, 101*(Suppl.), 1–12.

Yeagle, P. L. (1993). *The membranes of cells.* San Diego: Academic Press.

Zhao, H. B., Shellenberger, D. L., Shope, C. D., & Brownell, W. E. (2001). Cytoskeletal repair mechanisms in the outer hair cell lateral wall. *Abstracts of the Midwinter Research Meeting of the Association for Research in Otolaryngology, 24.*

Zheng, J., Shen, W., He, D. Z., Long, K. B., Madison, L. D., & Dallos, P. (2000). Prestin is the motor protein of cochlear outer hair cells. *Nature, 405*(6783), 149–155.

3

Mechanical Correlates of Fast Transducer Adaptation: Implications Toward Function and Underlying Mechanism

Anthony Ricci, PhD
Neuroscience Center of Excellence and Kresge Hearing Labs
Louisiana State University Health Sciences Center
New Orleans, Louisiana

MECHANOELECTRIC TRANSDUCTION

Hair cells are the mechanoreceptors of the inner ear. Specialized epithelial cells, hair cells have a tuft of stereocilia on their apical surface termed the hair bundle. The hair bundle contains the machinery for mechanoelectric transduction. Hair bundles are comprised of stereocilia, actin-filled projections that increase in height toward a tall end, where sometimes a true kinocilium is housed (Figure 3–1A) (Hackney, Fettiplace, & Furness, 1993; Tilney, DeRosier, & Mulroy, 1980; Tilney, Egelman, DeRosier, & Saunders, 1983; Tilney & DeRosier, 1986; Tilney & Saunders, 1983; Tilney, Tilney, Saunders, & DeRosier, 1986). The hair bundle is polarized so that deflection towards the tall edge opens mechanically gated channels, and deflection toward the short edge closes channels (Shotwell, Jacobs, & Hudspeth, 1981). Tip-links connect adjacent rows of stereocilia and define the axis of sensitivity for the hair bundle (Pickles et al., 1989). Examples of the tip-links can be seen in Figure 3–1. Tip-links are thought to deliver the mechanical stimulus to the transducer channels.

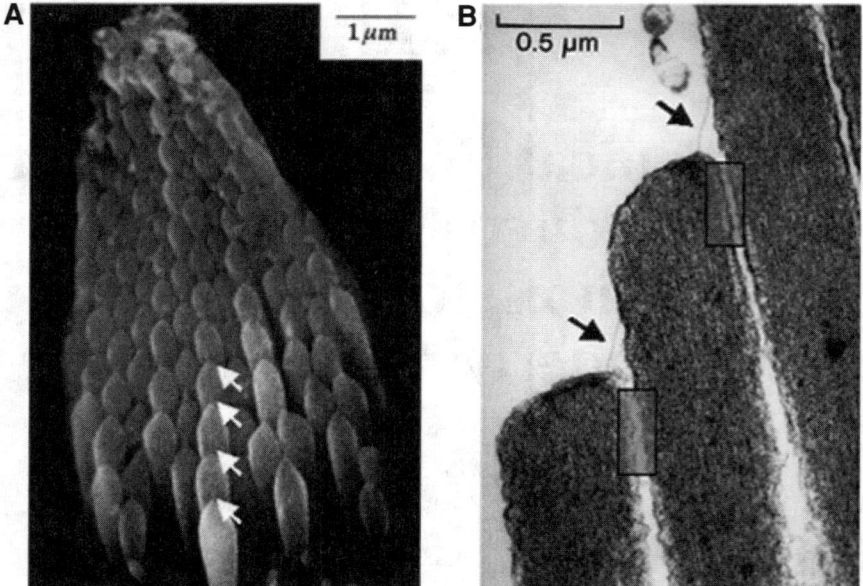

Figure 3–1. (**A**) Scanning electron micrograph of a hair bundle from a turtle auditory papilla hair cell. Note the increase in height of the stereocilia toward a tall edge. White arrows point to tip-links. Careful inspection shows the tip-links aligned in one direction. (**B**) Transmission electron micrograph of a cross-section of a hair bundle. Note the densely packed actin filaments. Black arrows point to tip-links. Debate remains as to the location of the transducer channels. Some data suggest the transducer channels are located at either or both ends of the tip-link. Other data postulate the channels are located at a site where the stereocilia come into close approximation. This area is shown in the boxes. Micrographs provided by David Furness and Carole Hackney.

Mechanoelectric transducer channels are located near the tops of the stereocilia (Denk, Holt, Shepherd, & Corey, 1995; Hudspeth, 1982; Jaramillo & Hudspeth, 1991; Lumpkin & Hudspeth, 1995). Debate remains, however, as to the exact location. Channels may be located at either or both ends of the tip-link. Data supporting this contention come from imaging stereociliary calcium with a two-photon system that allows high resolution of calcium changes (Denk et al., 1995). Data suggested that calcium changed at both the top of the shortest row of stereocilia, where there were no side links, as well as in the tallest row of stereocilia, where there were no top-links. The problem with this experiment is that it assumes the channels are at one location or the other, but the experiment does not test the validity of channels being located elsewhere near the tops of the stereocilia. Immunocyto-chemical evidence suggest the channels are located below the tip-link at a position where the stereocilia come close to each other (Figure 3–1B) (Hackney, Furness, Benos, Woodley, & Barratt, 1992; Furness, Hackney, & Benos, 1996). Antibodies to an amiloride sensitive channel labeled this region of the stereocilia. Amiloride and amiloride deriva-tives have previously been shown to block the transducer channel (Jorgensen & Ohmori, 1988; Rusch, Kros, & Richardson, 1994). Channels located at this region can also explain the calcium imaging experiments described previously. That is, signals would be measured in both the tallest and shortest stereocilia, respectively. The location of the channels has important implications as to the molecular mecha-nisms involved in the transduction process. For example, channels located at either end of the tip-links would be expected to show mechanical cooperativity. The location of the transducer channels also has implications regarding the mechanisms of adaptation.

The transducer channels are mechanically gated (Corey & Hudspeth, 1979; Hudspeth & Corey, 1977). The gating spring theory of channel activation suggests that force applied to the channels results in their opening (Figure 3–2). Opening of transducer channels leads to an increase in hair bundle compliance, typically rationalized as the activation gate being in series with a gating spring (Howard & Hudspeth, 1988). The idea is that the addition of the length of the channel gate increases bundle compliance. Transducer channels have been estimated to contribute between 35 and 80% of the hair bundle's compliance (Howard & Hudspeth, 1988; Marquis & Hudspeth, 1997). Nonlinearities in the force-displacement function have also been attributed to gating compliance (Howard & Hudspeth, 1988; Russell, Richardson, & Kossl, 1989). The gating compliance has been impli-cated as an important part of a mechanism responsible for generating mechanical oscillations of the hair bundle (Martin & Hudspeth, 1999; Martin, Mehta, & Hudspeth, 2000).

The transducer channel carries a nonselective cation current (Crawford, Evans, & Fettiplace, 1991; Jorgensen & Kroese, 1994, 1995; Lumpkin, Marquis, & Hudspeth, 1997; Ohmori, 1985, 1988; Ricci & Fettiplace, 1998). Calcium permeation through this channel regulates adaptation (Assad & Corey, 1992; Assad, Hacohen, & Corey, 1989; Crawford et al., 1991; Eatock, Corey, & Hudspeth, 1987; Hacohen, Assad, Smith, & Corey, 1989; Lumpkin et al., 1997; Marquis & Hudspeth, 1997; Ricci & Fettiplace, 1997, 1998; Ricci, Crawford, & Fettiplace, 2000; Ricci, Wu, & Fettiplace, 1998; van Netten & Kros,

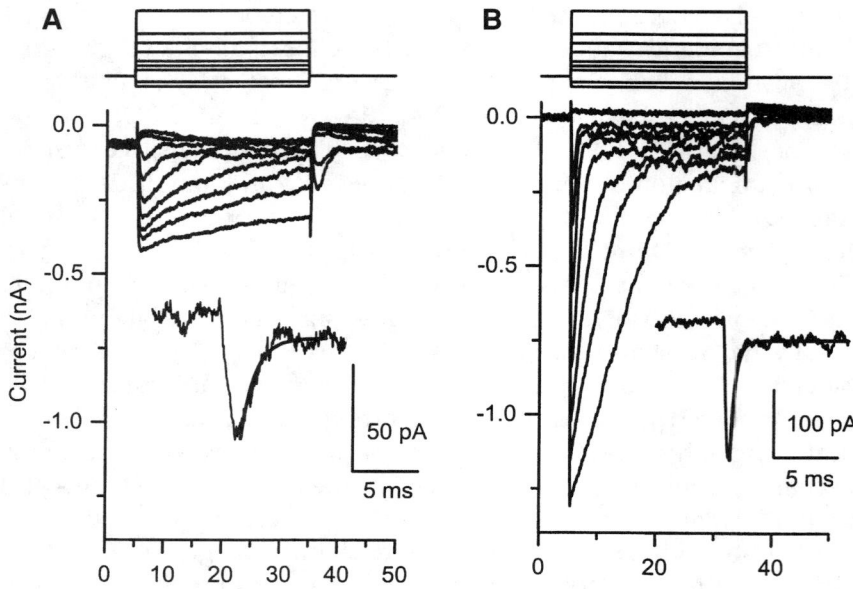

Figure 3–2. Examples of transducer currents recorded from turtle auditory papilla hair cells. (**A**) is a low-frequency hair cell (~0.3 relative distance from lagena), and (**B**) is a high-frequency hair cell (~0.65 relative distance from lagena). The use of the intact preparation allows for tonotopic variations to be measured. The cells were voltage-clamped at −80mV, and the currents measured were in response to mechanical deflections of the hair bundle (stimuli shown above current records). Positive stimuli indicate toward the kinocilium, opening channels; negative stimuli indicate away from the kinocilium, closing channels. Adaptation is seen in both hair cells as a decrease in current during a constant stimulus. Note how fast and complete adaptation is for small deflections of the hair bundle. The insets are expansions of the hair cell's response to a small deflection. The solid lines represent single exponential fits to the decay in the current records, with time constants of 2 and 0.75 ms, respectively.

2000; Wu, Ricci, & Fettiplace, 1999). Adaptation manifests itself as a decrease in current during a constant stimulus (Figure 3–3). Recent evidence suggests that adaptation is a complex process involving multiple mechanisms (Wu et al., 1999). At least two independent components of adaptation have been identified based on kinetics, pharmacology, and operating range (Wu et al., 1999). The purpose of this chapter is to review the data regarding the functional role of adaptation as well as to provide information regarding mechanical correlates of adaptation and their implications regarding the molecular mechanism of adaptation.

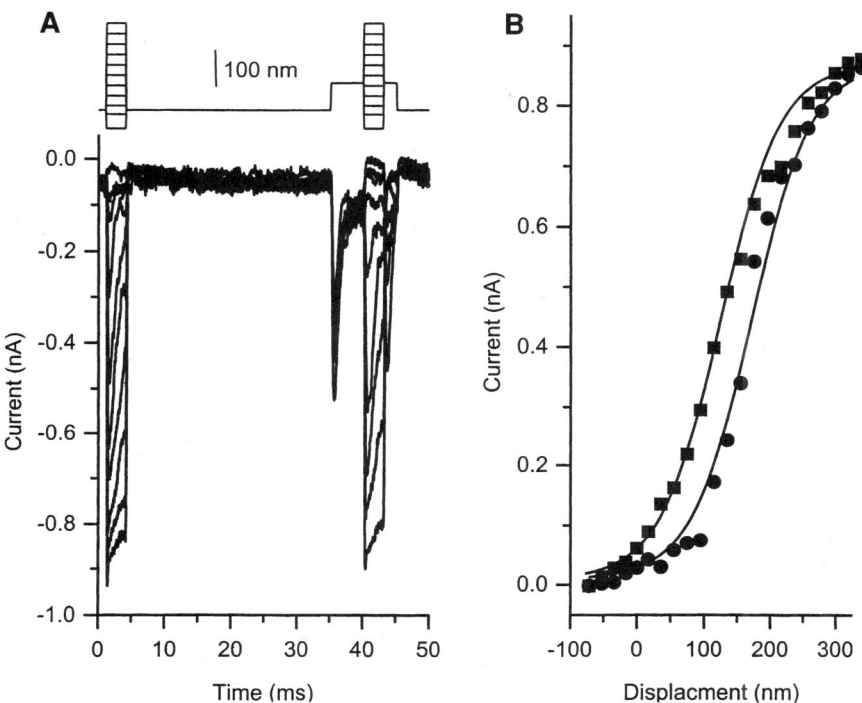

Figure 3–3. Adaptation is classically thought of as shifting in the activation curve of the transducer channels. The protocol and currents elicited by a protocol intended to demonstrate this shift are given in (**A**). Activation curves are plotted for the peak currents elicited from a series of mechanical deflections about the cells' resting bundle position or following an adaptive step (**B**). The activation curve shifts about 50 nm to the right in response to a 75 nm adaptive bundle deflection, suggesting for this cell that adaptation was not complete. Single Boltzmann functions were fit to each plot, demonstrating a shift in the half activation point but no change in either the slope or the maximal current. The cell was voltage-clamped at −80mV.

METHODS

Data presented in this chapter come from recordings made in the intact auditory papilla of the turtle *Trachemys scripta elegans*, the red-eared slider. All animal protocols were approved by the Animal Care Utilization Community (ACUC) at Louisiana State University (LSU) Health Sciences Center. The methods used for isolating and recording from this preparation have been detailed elsewhere (Ricci & Fettiplace, 1997). Whole-cell recordings were used to voltage-clamp (holding potential was −80 mV) hair cells in order to electrically isolate the mechanically gated channel. The turtle auditory papilla is tono-topically organized (Crawford & Fettiplace, 1980; Ricci, Gray-Keller & Fettiplace, 2000). By advancing the recording electrodes perpendicular to the tonotopic axis, it was possible to select a particular frequency range to explore. Glass probes attached to a piezo-electric device were used to mechanically stimulate the hair bundle (Figure 3–4). Either stiff probes, where the probe is much stiffer than the hair bundle, or flexible fibers, where the probe is approximately equivalent to the hair bundle stiffness, were used to deliver displacement or force steps, respectively (Crawford & Fettiplace, 1985). Fiber stiffness was cali-brated by measuring, with a horizontal microscope, the deflection of the fiber produced by hanging polymethylmethacrylate beads on its tip (Howard & Ashmore, 1986; Ricci, Crawford, et al., 2000).

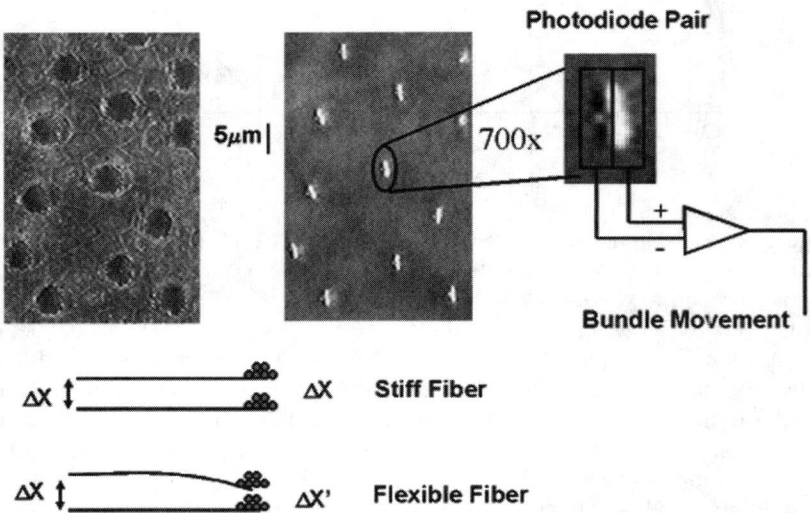

Figure 3–4. A schematic of the methods used for stimulating the hair bundle as well as for imaging hair bundle movements. Two Nomarski images show the base of the hair bundles (left) and the tops of the hair bundles (right). Individual cilia and the tops of the supporting cells can be seen in the left panel. The light piping ability of the hair bundle can be seen on the right. Projecting the bright hair bundle image onto a pair of differentially amplified photodiodes (far right) at a magnification of 700x allowed for the direct measurement of hair bundle movements. Lower schematic represents the types of stimuli applied to the hair bundles. Stiff fibers moved the hair bundles as far as the probe was displaced. Flexible fibers allowed the hair bundle to move the probe by a distance that was related to the force applied to the bundle and to the stiffness of the hair bundle.

The stiffness of the fibers ranged between 0.5 and 1.5 mN/m. Motion of the hair bundle was measured by projecting the image of the hair bundle onto a pair of differentially amplified photodiodes. Taking advantage of the hair bundle's ability to light pipe and thereby provide a bright line of light allows for the direct imaging of the hair bundle. Direct imaging of the hair bundle is an advantage over previous experiments where a stimulating probe was imaged (Crawford & Fettiplace, 1985; Howard & Ashmore, 1986). Imaging the bundle allowed for free-standing bundle movements elicited by depolarization to be measured. In addition, imaging allows for flexible fibers to be constructed that are quite fast. It was no longer necessary to construct a probe of dimensions that would image well. That is, the probe could be shorter and thinner than in previous experiments, thereby limiting viscous drag and allowing for faster rise times of the stimulus. Fast rise times were imperative for the maintenance of fast adaptation (Wu et al., 1999). The stimulus rise time in the experiments reported here was approximately 150 μs. The stiffness of the hair bundle was directly assessed by knowing the stiffness of the fiber (Kf), the position of the fiber on the hair bundle (λ, fractional distance from top of bundle), the measured movement of the hair bundle (x), and the known displacement of the fixed end of the probe (z). The stiffness of the bundle Kb is then estimated as:

$$Kb = Kf^* \lambda^2 (z - \lambda x)/\lambda x$$

All data were sampled at 10–40 kHz using a CED (Cambridge Electronic Devices) and accompanying software. Series resistance varied from 3 to 20 MΩ and was compensated 50–75%. Cell capacitance ranged from 8–17 pF.

CLASSICAL ADAPTATION

Classically, adaptation has been thought of as a means of preventing saturation by shifting the operating range of the transducer channels (Figure 3–3) (Eatock et al., 1987; Crawford, Evans, & Fettiplace, 1989). Shifting the operating range of the transducer channel also serves to maintain sensitivity and possibly prevent hair bundle damage. In this light, adaptation is a steady-state phenomenon, the kinetics of which have been largely ignored. Classical adaptation typically had time constants, measured from the decay in current during a constant stimulus, in the tens of milliseconds (Burlacu, Tap, Lumpkin, & Husapeth, 1997; Eatock et al., 1987; Gillespie & Hudspeth, 1993; Holt, Corey, & Eatock, 1997; Howard & Hudspeth, 1987; Roberts, Howards & Hudspeth, 1988; Shepherd & Corey, 1994). Classical adaptation is postulated to be a decrease in hair bundle stiffness imparted by a myosin isozyme (Gillespie, 1997; Gillespie & Corey, 1997; Howard & Hudspeth, 1987; Steyger, Gillespie, & Baird, 1998; Wolfrum, Liu, Schmitt, Udovichenko, & Williams, 1998). The myosin isozyme is thought to link the transducer channels to the cytoskeleton. Calcium entry through the transducer channel is thought to cause myosin to "slip" along the actin filaments, reducing tension in the hair bundle closing channels. Channel closure, which reduces calcium in the stereocilia, would cause myosin to climb the actin filament, increasing tension in the hair bundle opening transducer channels. A variety of data support this form of adaptation. Antagonists of myosin shift the activation curve rightward (Gillespie & Hudspeth, 1993; Yamoah & Gillespie, 1996). Voltage-dependent movements of the hair bundle have been monitored. The myosin model predicts that lowering stereocilia calcium by depolarization causes the motors to climb the stereocilia, moving the hair bundle away from the tall edge. This result was observed in frog saccule hair cells (Assad et al., 1989). Measurements of bundle compliance also suggested that the hair bundle became less stiff during hair bundle deflection (Howard & Hudspeth, 1987). It should be noted that transducer currents were not measured simultaneously during these experiments, and other investigators have demonstrated an uncoupling between adaptation and a time-dependent increase in hair bundle compliance (Kros, 1995). The motor was determined to be near the transducer channels, based on experiments that first removed adaptation by depolarization and then measured the time to recovery of adaptation. A time course of 2 ms was noted which, based on diffusion models, suggested the motor must be within a micrometer of the channel (Assad et al., 1989). With the discovery of a second, faster component of adaptation, this result may be open for reinterpretation. Immunocytochemical experiments demonstrate myosin 1B labeling along the sides and at the tops of stereocilia, locations presumably appropriate for the motor model of adaptation (Garcia, Yee, Gillespie, & Corey, 1998; Gillespie, Wagner, & Hudspeth, 1993; Metcalf, Chelliah, & Hudspeth, 1994; Steyger et al., 1998). A necklace of staining was also found in the cuticular plate region.

The motor model of adaptation typically puts the transducer channels at either end of the tip-links and has the channels moving along the sides of the stereocilia during adaptation. One result of this configuration would have the channels on the sides dictating adaptation to the channels at both ends of the link. If the motors were at the top of the stereocilia, slipping would be ineffective at reducing tension because reducing tension in the link would require the channel to move up the stereocilia. To increase tension, myosin would be required to climb down the stereocilia; this is unlikely, due to the orientation of the actin. These constraints suggest that the motor component of adaptation be applicable to channels located on the sides of the stereocilia, and not those located on the top. If the channels are located below the tip-links at the region where the stereocilia are in close proximity, then the organization of the motors would again have to be different. Motors could be present on either side of the membrane, and channels could move in either direction but the extent of travel would be limited by the distance of close apposition between the two membranes. On the other hand, the channel may sense force exerted between the surface membrane and the cytoskeleton. In this way, the channel does not have to move up or down the stereocilia at all. The problem with this possibility is that the immunocytochemistry suggests the myosin is not localized to this location. In fact, at the moment, a dichotomy exists in the literature: the localization of the myosin responsible for force generation does not correlate with the localization of the channel. As described above, localization of myosin does not completely correspond to the motor theory of adaptation.

FAST ADAPTATION AS A TUNING MECHANISM

The development of intact preparations for investigating mechano-electric transduction processes has allowed for more detailed investigations than previously possible (Geleoc, Lennan, Richardson, & Kros, 1997; Holt et al., 1997; Kros, Rusch, & Richardson, 1992; Ricci & Fettiplace, 1997). In particular, it has allowed for investigation into tonotopic differences in transduction (Ricci & Fettiplace, 1997). In turtle auditory papilla, a fast component of adaptation has been described (Figures 3–3 and 3–4) (Crawford et al., 1989, 1991; Ricci & Fettiplace, 1997, 1998; Ricci et al., 1998). The rate of fast adaptation varied tonotopically, with time constants ranging from 3 ms at the low frequency end to less than 1 ms at the higher frequencies (Fettiplace & Fuchs, 1999; Ricci & Fettiplace, 1997). The fastest time constants measured were comparable to the rise time of the stimulus, near 100 μsec.

First observations demonstrated that the rate of adaptation varied with the characteristic frequency and tonotopic organization of the auditory papilla. This correlation suggested that adaptation might serve as a high pass filter to acoustic input (Ricci & Fettiplace, 1997). Alone, this filtering role would be novel and understanding the mechanism important. Further investigations revealed that transducer currents could undergo damped oscillations (Ricci et al., 1998). The oscillations were calcium-dependent and most prevalent at endolymphatic levels of calcium (Figure 3–5) (Ricci et al., 1998). Endolymph is the solution bathing the apical hair bundles; it is unusual in that it has a high potassium concentration and a low micromolar calcium concentration (Bosher & Warren, 1978). The frequency of the oscillations varied tonotopically. Fast adaptation appears to underlie in part the tonotopic transducer current oscillations (Ricci et al., 1998; Wu et al., 1999). The presence of the oscillations has led to the hypothesis that adaptation, particularly fast adaptation, serves as an amplification and filtering mechanism for hair cells (Ricci et al., 1998; Wu et al., 1999). Similar arguments have been made for frog saccule hair cells where damped oscillations of lower frequencies have been observed (Benser, Marquis, & Hudspeth, 1996). Although here a link to a second component of adaptation has not been made.

If the transducer current oscillations are present in mammalian systems, they may underlie at least part of the active process. The active process provides amplification needed for the mammalian cochlea to achieve measured sensitivities. The passive traveling wave of vonBekesy is thought to be boosted by an electromechanical amplification process. To date the active process has largely been attributed to outer hair cell (OHC) motility (Nobili, Mammano, & Ashmore, 1998). The OHC acts as both sensor and feedback control. Several lines of evidence suggest that more than OHC motility is required. First, data above demonstrate the existence of a mechanical filtering mechanism in the hair bundle. As demonstrated in the following, a mechanical correlate exists for fast adaptation and suggests an active force-generating system is involved. Second, otoacoustic emissions, typically thought to be a by-product of the active process, have been identified in species that do not have OHCs (Koppl & Manley, 1993; Probst, Lonsbury-Martin, & Martin, 1991; Stewart & Hudspeth, 2000). These emissions show a similar pharmacological sensitivity to those produced in mammalian cochleae (Brown, McDowell, & Forge, 1989; Stewart & Hudspeth, 2000). Finally, modeling work has demonstrated the feasibility of hair bundle movements accounting for at least part of

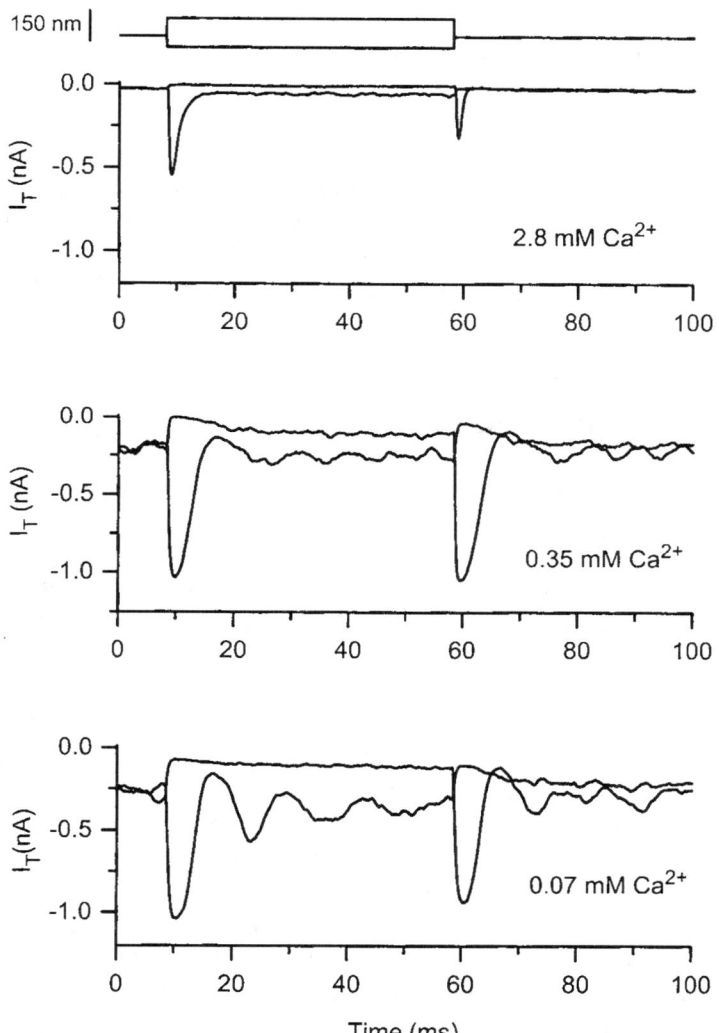

Figure 3–5. Transducer currents (below) and mechanical stimuli (above) are given for an individual hair cell while changing the external calcium concentrations from 2.8 mM to 0.35 mM to 0.07 mM, respectively. Adaptation was fast, but no hint of oscillations could be observed in the high calcium concentration. As external calcium was lowered the transducer currents became larger, due to the release of a calcium block of the channel; the magnitude of current on at rest was increased, due to an adaptive shift in the activation curve; and a robust oscillation in the transducer current could be observed. The oscillation was observed for positive deflections of the hair bundle as well as during the recovery of a negative deflection of the hair bundle.

the active process (Markin & Hudspeth, 1995b; Martin & Hudspeth, 1999). Understanding the mechanism of fast adaptation is important because it may underlie in part the active process. Quantitating the force generated by adaptation as well as the kinetic limitations of the process will aid in our better understanding of the initial steps of signal transduction in the ear. Fast adaptation per se may be a misnomer. The functional significance of the processes underlying fast adaptation may be more relevant as regards tuning and amplification than toward maintaining sensitivity or extending the dynamic range of the cell.

DISTINGUISHING FAST ADAPTATION FROM CLASSICAL ADAPTATION

Fast adaptation has been suggested to be a separate entity from the classical motor model of adaptation based on several pieces of evidence. First, the kinetics of adaptation are faster than any measured kinetics for a myosin isozyme, particularly myosin 1B or myosin VIIa (Ricci & Fettiplace, 1997, 1998; Wu et al., 1999). Second, the decay of the current during a constant stimulus follows a double exponential time course for all but the smallest stimuli (Wu et al., 1999). The relative proportion of the fast and slow component varies with stimulus intensities, with the slow component becoming more prominent for larger deflections. Finally, myosin ATPase antagonists previously reported to inhibit adaptation by interfering with the motor process do not block the fast component of adaptation (Yamoah & Gillespie, 1996; Wu et al., 1999). The activation curve does shift, but this may be due to calcium loading (a result of antagonizing the stereociliary CaATPases) as much as due to the blocking of the motor. Although these data are compelling, they leave something to be desired in that they are indirect assessments. To more directly address the underlying changes in hair bundle mechanics associated with fast adaptation, experiments were designed to measure hair bundle movements and the forces generated by the hair bundle.

VOLTAGE-DEPENDENT HAIR BUNDLE MOVEMENTS

Depolarization to potentials near +80mV reduces the driving force for calcium entry through transduction channels. The transducer current becomes outward. Stereociliary calcium is reduced, triggering an adaptive response. The motor model suggests that the motor will climb along the actin filaments up the stereocilia, increasing tension in the tip-links and opening channels.

This hypothesis suggests and data support the conclusion that the hair bundle will move away from the tall edge toward the short edge of the stereocilia (Assad et al., 1989). An alternate hypothesis that treats adaptation as a calcium-dependent feedback system suggests that lowering calcium in the stereocilia will result in the opening of transducer channels and the bundle moving toward the kinocilium or tall edge of the hair bundle as a result of the channel opening (Crawford et al., 1991; Wu et al., 1999). Experiments to test this hypothesis have been performed, and an example of the results is given in Figure 3–6. Upon depolarization, the transducer current turns on, shifting the activation curve to the right in an attempt to restore calcium homeostasis. Concomitant with the transducer current turning on is a rapid movement of the hair bundle toward the kinocilium. This motion is opposite that predicted by the motor model of adaptation. A small rapid step in movement away from the kinocilia was also observed during depolarization. This movement was not dependent on the transducer channel or on calcium and so is not being analyzed in detail at this time. It does not appear to be related to adaptation (see Ricci, Crawford, et al., 2000, for details). Holding the hair bundle in place with a stiff probe during the depolarizing step (Figure 3–6) could block both the current turning on and the hair bundle movement. The kinetics of the current turning on were complex and probably related to the dissipation of a calcium gradient in the stereocilia (Ricci et al., 1998). Nonetheless, in both the current onset and hair bundle movement, the rise time could be fit with an exponential.

A plot of the time constant measured for the current onset against the time constant for the movement onset demonstrates a good correlation (Figure 3–7). The slope of one and intercept of zero indicates that the movement and channel opening occur simultaneously. This too is opposed to predictions by the motor model that suggest the bundle move first and then the channels respond to the change in force being exerted. The similarity in time constant suggests a much more intimate association between channel state and bundle movement.

A second piece of information gathered from these data is the relationship between transducer current magnitude and the magnitude of the hair bundle movement. If the movement is dictated by a process intimately associated with the channel, then a direct correlation can be drawn between hair bundle movement and number of transducer channels.

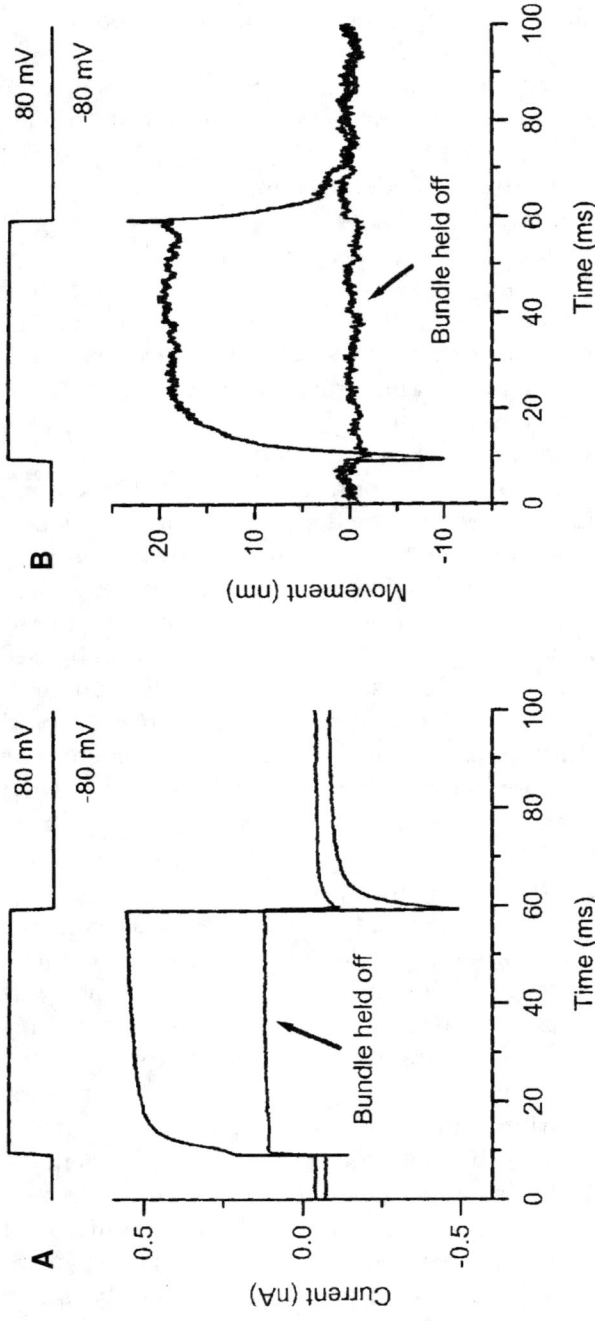

Figure 3-6. (A) Transducer current response to depolarization from −80mV to +80 mV. The transducer current turns on and appears as an outward current during depolarization. Both an instantaneous component and increasing current can be observed. At the offset two components of decay can be seen in the tail response. When a stiff probe is used to hold the hair bundle off, no current turns on in response to depolarization. The tail response is also significantly reduced. **(B)** The hair bundle movement in response to depolarization from −80mV to +80 mV. A rapid step movement away from the kinocilium, is observed followed by a movement toward the kinocilium. The movement shows similar kinetics to the current. The initial apparent transient response was not dependent on transducer channels or upon external calcium and so is not interpreted as being a component of adaptation. When a stiff probe is held against the bundle, no movements were observed. The polarity of this movement was opposite that reported in frog saccule cells where a motor model of adaptation was used to describe the phenomenon.

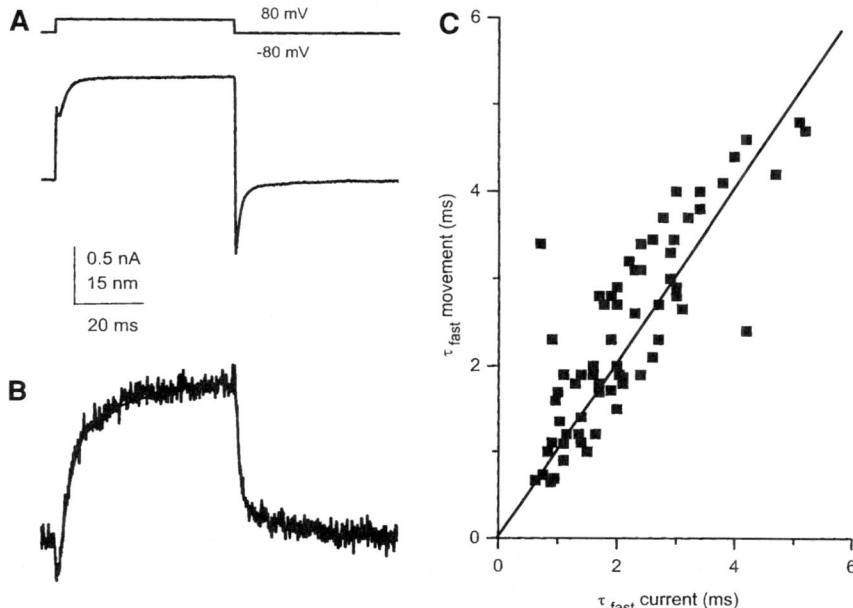

Figure 3–7. (**A**) Upper panels illustrate the transducer currents response to depolarization from –80 mV to +80mV. The stimulus time-course is given at the top of the panel. A single exponential could be fit to the time course of the current onset. (**B**) A plot of hair bundle movement in response to the same depolarization. Here too a single exponential could be fit to the rise time of the bundle movement. (**C**) A plot of the time constant of the hair bundle movement (τ_m) against the time constant for the current onset (τ_I). The solid line represents a slope of one and an intercept of zero. The plot suggests that the current onset and hair bundle movement occur simultaneously.

On the other hand, a motor system can have any number of motors associated with the transducer channel, and this number might vary, so the relationship between current size and bundle movement need not be direct. Figure 3–8 plots transducer current size against hair bundle movement, demonstrating a direct linear relationship. An example of how the measurements were made is given in part A of Figure 3–7.

Additional information can be gleaned from these data. Although as mentioned, interpreting the onset kinetics with depolarization is complex, it is possible to evaluate the offsets. Repolarization from 80 mV to –80 mV restores the driving force for calcium. Open transducer channels will now close as calcium rushes in. The corresponding tail current follows an exponential time course as do the corresponding

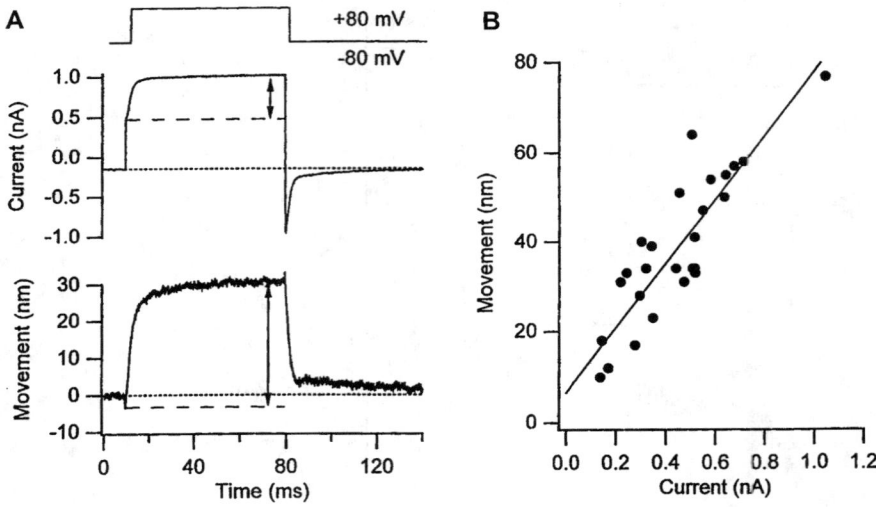

Figure 3–8. (A) Upper panel shows transducer current response to depolarization from –80mV to +80mV. The arrows indicate how the magnitude of the transducer current was measured. Lower panel illustrates the hair bundle movement in response to the same depolarization. Here too the arrows indicates how the magnitude of the movement was measured. A plot of the peak movement versus the peak current shows a good correlation (r = 0.89). The data suggest that the number of transducer channels present directly dictates the magnitude of the bundle movement. The motor model of adaptation does not support this result where the number of motors would dictate the movement. The result does suggest a more intimate relationship between the transducer channels and fast adaptation as represented by the hair bundle movement.

tails of the movement. Examples of these tail responses are shown in Figure 3–8. Good correlations can be found by plotting the time constants obtained from the currents against those of the movements (data not shown, see Ricci, Crawford, et al., 2000). However, is it more important to evaluate the relationships of time constants of the hair bundle movement or the time constants of adaptation obtained from hair bundle deflections? That is, we can use the correlation between the double exponential fits to the current decay in response to a step deflection of the hair bundle and the double exponential decay of the hair bundle movement in response to a repolarization from 80 mV to –80 mV as an assessment of whether we are investigating a similar phenomenon under these two very different experimental conditions. Figure 3–9 plots these results, and there is a good correlation between

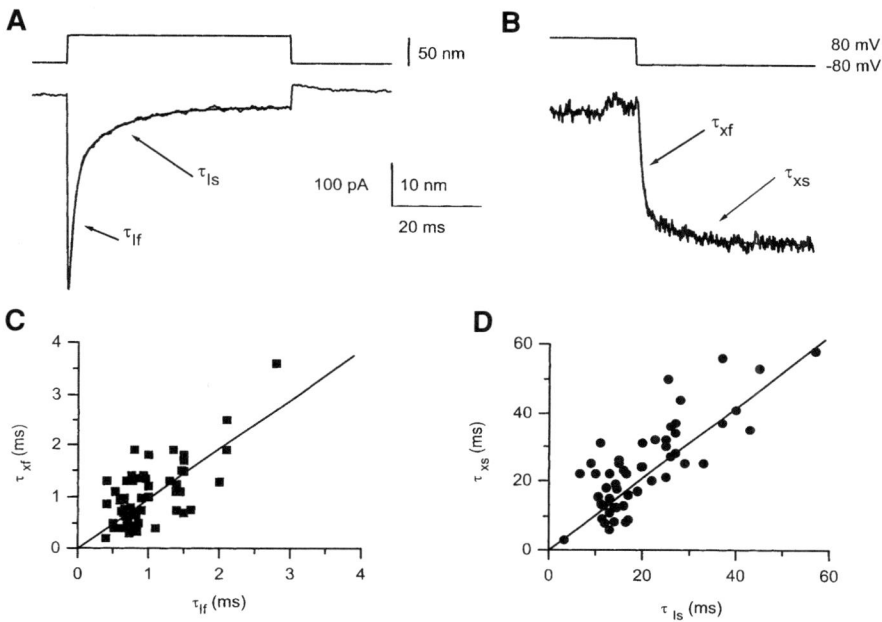

Figure 3–9. (**A**) Response of a hair cell to a 50 nm deflection of the hair bundle. The transducer current shows a robust adaptation whose decay can best be fit by the sum of two exponentials. Fast and slow time constants (τ_{if} and τ_{is}) can be derived from these fits. The fit is shown as the solid line. The scale bar is given in the center and the stimulus shown above for both (**A & B**). The hair cell was voltage-clamped at –80mV for the experiment. (**B**) The mechanical response of a hair bundle upon repolarization from +80 mV to –80 mV. The decay in the movement could also be best fit by the sum of two exponentials from which two time constants, a fast (τ_{xf}) and a slow (τ_{xs}) could be derived. Plotting the corresponding fast time constants (τ_{xf} vs. τ_{if}) in (**C**) and slow time constants (τ_{xs} vs. τ_{is}) (**D**) give reasonably good correlations between currents and movements. These results demonstrate that at least kinetically a similar mechanism underlies the two manifestations of transducer adaptation.

the fast and slow time constants in current and movement measured in the same cell by these two different protocols. The good correlations demonstrate that the processes being investigated by these two disparate methods most likely arise from a common mechanism.

Together, the results from the voltage induced hair bundle movements suggest that fast adaptation does not occur by the classical motor model for adaptation. They suggest there is a mechanical component to fast adaptation, and it is a force-generating process since it takes force to open the transducer channels. Also, the data suggest a tight coupling between the state of the transducer channel and the motion of the hair bundle.

MECHANICAL CORRELATE OF FAST ADAPTATION

Characterizing the mechanical properties of the hair bundle elicited by fast adaptation is important because it will give insight into the mechanisms underlying the process. In addition, a mechanical correlate of fast adaptation is predicted if fast adaptation underlies a component of the active process. Stimulating the hair bundle with a flexible fiber approximates force steps to the hair bundle. Bundle movements in response to force stimuli were measured with the photodiode. The flexible fiber allows the hair bundle to move independently of the stimulus applied.

Figure 3–10 presents representative examples of hair cell responses to small force displacements for high-frequency cells. The bundle movement was a mirror image of the transducer current. The first point noted is that the bundle movement during adaptation suggests an increase in hair bundle stiffness. That is, for the same force step the bundle is moving less during and following adaptation than before adapting. This polarity of movement is opposite that reported for motor-based adaptation. The simplest interpretation of this data is that the bundle is getting stiffer and that a counter force is being exerted to oppose bundle movement. A second piece of information that can be obtained from these data is that the kinetics of the movement correlates with the time course of the current. Plotting the time constant of the transducer current decay against the time constant of the movement (Figure 3–11) demonstrates a linear relationship. The solid line has a slope of one and intercept of zero. The dashed line is the linear regression fit to the data.

Conservatively, the data suggest that the current and movement occur simultaneously. At the very least, the data do not support the argument that the movement would occur first. The motor model of adaptation would have the movement occurring prior to the channel gating, with the movement resulting in channel closure. The data do not support the motor model. If the regression fit data are correct, the data suggest the movement occurred after the channel had closed as a result of channel closing. Similar types of hair bundle movements have been observed in frog saccule cells (Benser et al., 1996; Howard

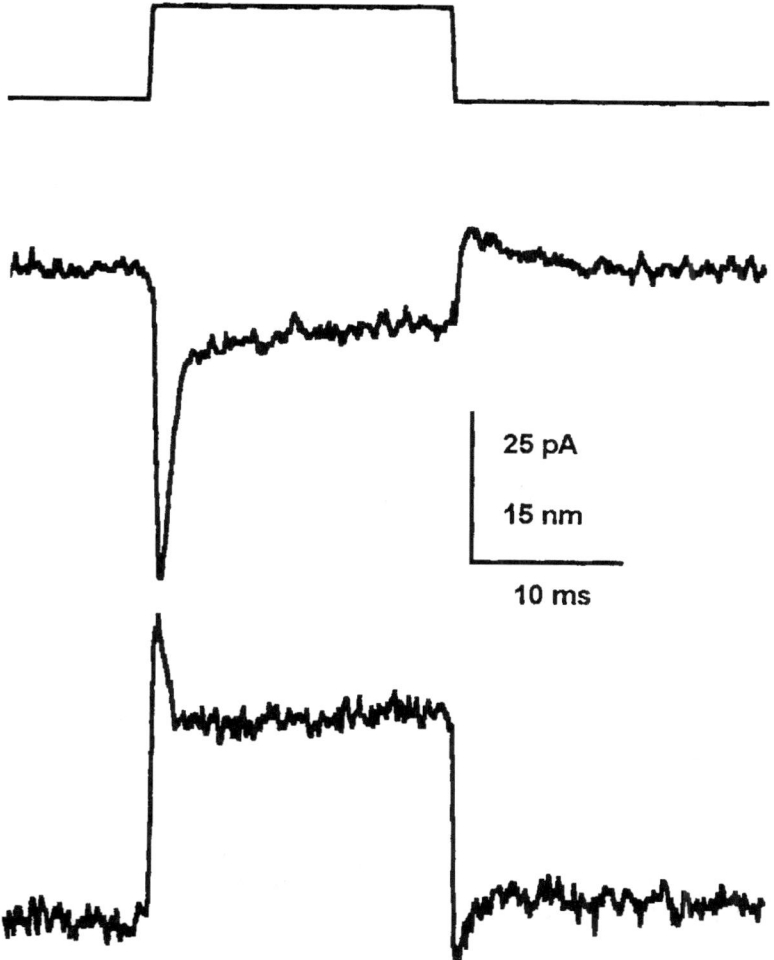

Figure 3–10. Example of a transducer current and hair bundle response to a flexible fiber stimulus. The stimulus time-course is given above the responses. The current onset is fast as is adaptation, demonstrating the fast rise time of the probe. The hair cell was voltage-clamped at –80 mV for the experiment. The movement is virtually a mirror image of the transducer current. A rapid, apparent increase in hair bundle stiffness is observed to correlate with adaptation. This result is counter to that predicted by the motor model of adaptation where the hair bundle should become more compliant during adaptation; thus, the movement would be predicted to continue further toward the kinocilium as opposed to reversing direction and moving away from the kinocilium. Time constants could be derived from single exponential fits to the decay in the current and in the movement. The solid lines represent the fits.

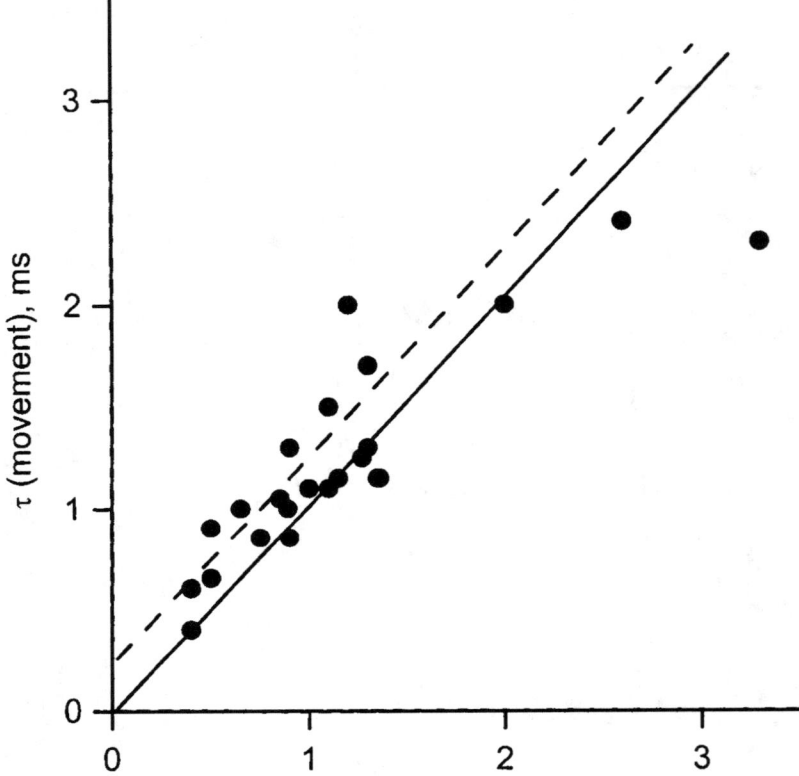

Figure 3–11. Time constants could be derived for both the adaptation seen in the current as well as the adaptation observed in the hair bundle movement. A plot of the time constant derived from the movements against the time constants derived from the currents is shown. The solid line represents a slope of one and an intercept of zero. The dashed line represents a delay of 0.2 ms between the current onset and movement. These data would suggest that the channel closes and then the bundle moves in response to the closure. This interpretation is also different than would be predicted by the motor model of adaptation. The motor model suggests the bundle movement would precede the change in transducer current and that the channels close in response to the bundle movement relieving tension.

& Hudspeth, 1987). In each case, however, the correlation with a fast adaptation process was not clear.

If the bundle movement measured is a result of fast adaptation, then it should have properties similar to those of adaptation. For example, the movements should slow when external calcium is lowered.

The movements should also slow if the cell is depolarized, lowering the driving force for calcium entry. Figure 3–12A is an example of a cell's response at different holding potentials. As predicted, the bundle movements slow as adaptation is slowed. Similar bundle movement responses were seen, albeit slower, in frog saccule hair cells (Benser et al., 1996). A summary plot of a compilation of cells where adaptation was slowed either by depolarization or by lowering external calcium is given in Figure 3–12b. The plot of the time constants for the current decay against the movement decay is linear, with a slope of one and an intercept of zero.

Fast adaptation is most prevalent for small displacements eliciting less than 50% of the maximal current. Similarly, the hair bundle movements associated with fast adaptation are most robust for small displacements. Figure 3–13 is an example of a hair cell's response to a series of increasing force steps. The current-displacement plot demonstrates that fast adaptation and the corresponding bundle movements are most prevalent during the steepest portion of the activation curve. The force-displacement plot for this cell is also informative. A nonlinearity exists at the steepest portion of the activation curve. This is also where adaptation is the most robust. The nonlinearity is a demonstration of the gating theory of activation where channel opening increases hair bundle compliance (Howard & Hudspeth, 1988). The hair bundle stiffness can be modeled as the difference between a linear passive component and a nonlinear active component. The passive component represents the ankle stiffness, and the active component is contributed by channel gating and represented by a Boltzmann function. When all the channels are closed, the force displacement function is linear, with the slope equivalent to the passive stiffness. When all the channels are open, the force displacement plot is also linear, with the slope also equivalent to the passive stiffness. Two identical lines, having the same Y-intercept, would signify that the channel gating does not alter hair bundle compliance. The rightward shift in the linear component and the extent of this shift represents the channel contribution to hair bundle compliance. The transition from one line, where the channels are closed, to the other, where channels are open, can be represented by a Boltzmann function derived from the activation curve for the channel. The presence of the nonlinearity in the force displacement plot and the fact that the nonlinearity corresponds to the steepest portion of the activation curve therefore corroborates the gating spring theory of channel activation and demonstrates that the transducer channels contribute to the hair bundle compliance.

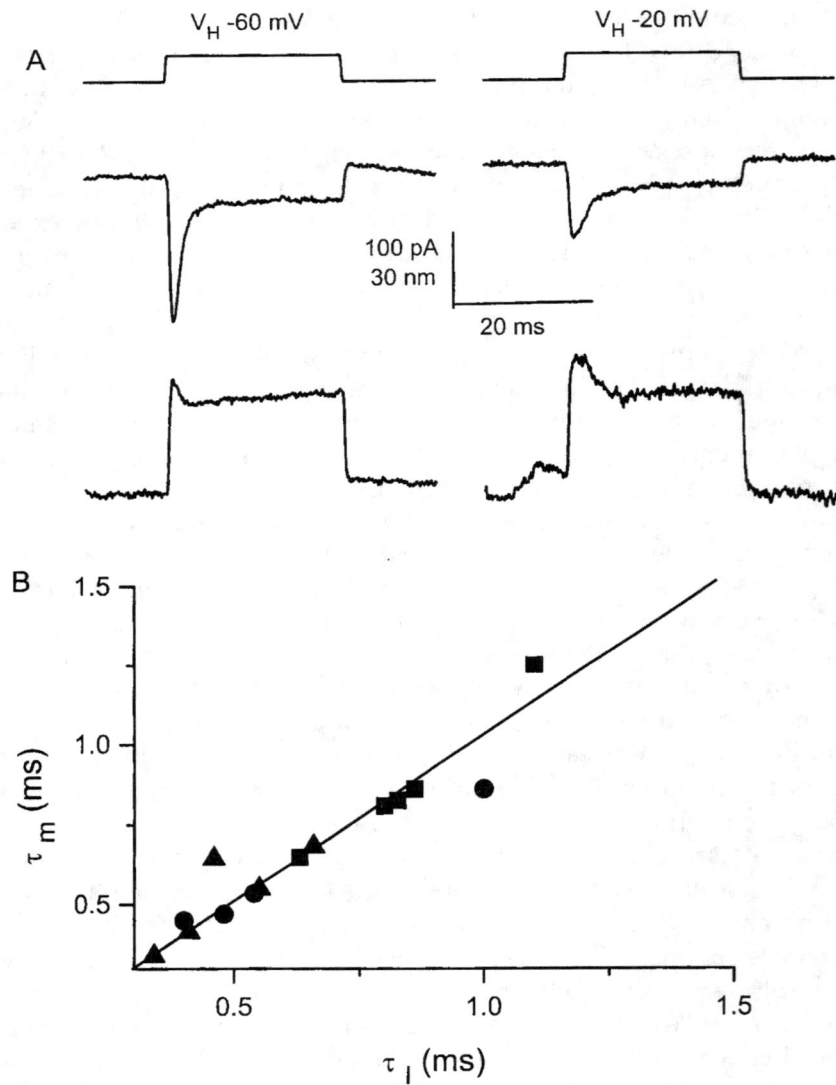

Figure 3–12. (**A**) Example of transducer currents and hair bundle movements in response to deflection with a flexible fiber. The hair cell was voltage-clamped at either –60 mV (left) or –20 mV (right). Adaptation slows when the cell is depolarized, presumably due to decreasing the driving force for calcium entry. (**B**) A summary plot where the time constants of the adaptation measured in the hair bundle movement is plotted against the current time constant under conditions that alter the calcium driving force, either depolarization or lowering external calcium levels. The line indicates a slope of one and an intercept of zero. Different symbols indicate different cells.

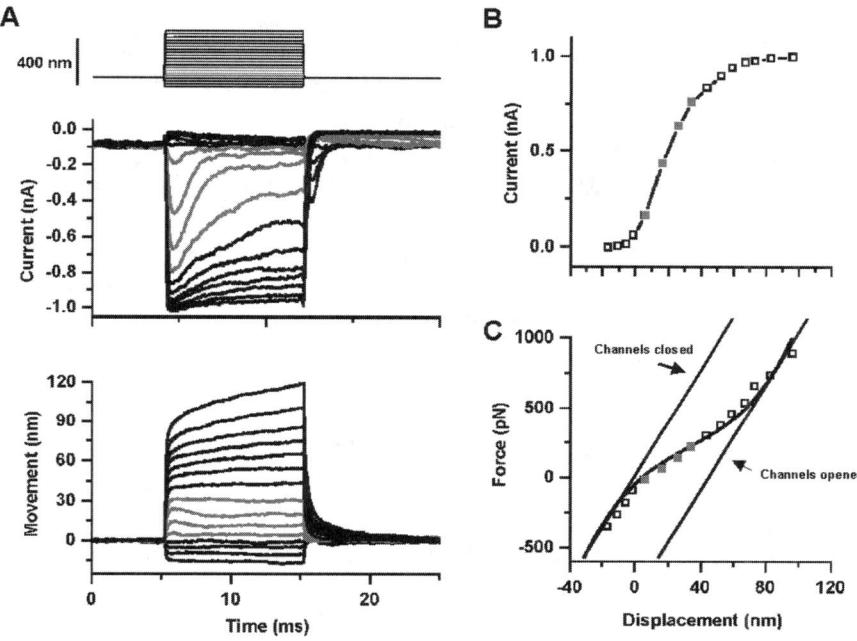

Figure 3–13. (**A**) Upper panes indicate stimuli time course and relative amplitude of force steps applied to a hair bundle. The transducer currents (middle)
and hair bundle movements (bottom) demonstrate that fast adaptation and the
corresponding hair bundle movements occur for stimuli eliciting less than 50%
of the maximal response. The current-displacement curve (**B**) shows that fast
adaptation occurs during the steepest portion of the activation curve (filled symbols). Force-displacement plot is shown in (**C**). Fast adaptation occurs during the
nonlinear portion of the curve. The shape of this curve supports the gating
spring theory of channel activation. The solid line represents the difference
between a line and a Boltzmann function, derived from the activation curve.
Data suggest that fast adaptation is intimately associated with the transducer
channel state (see text for details).

If adaptation is a parallel shift in the activation curve, then it can
be surmised that the passive properties of the hair bundle do not
change nor does the contribution to compliance by the channels. This
being the case, the linear components of the force-displacement plot
should not change during adaptation. The only change will be the
position of the nonlinear (Boltzmann function) component of the plot.
It is possible then to imagine that the bundle movement corresponding to the fast component of adaptation represents shifting of
the nonlinear component of the force-displacement function. This

interpretation would not require a change in hair bundle compliance. It should be remembered that the voltage-dependent hair bundle movements suggest a force-generating adaptation mechanism.

Together, the data pertaining to active bundle movements and fast adaptation demonstrate that fast adaptation is not equivalent to the motor model of adaptation. Fast adaptation appears to be tightly associated with the state of the transducer channel. An active force-generating system is postulated to be involved, though no compliance change is required to account for the reported data. Although the mechanical correlate of adaptation varies tonotopically, it is unclear what underlies these variations.

FUTURE DIRECTIONS

Data presented demonstrate that a rapid hair bundle movement occurs corresponding to the fast component of adaptation. The ability of the hair bundle to move rapidly suggests it can be a candidate for the active process in mammailian hair cells. Oscillations of the hair bundle have been observed and modeled where the underlying mechanisms appears to involve the interaction of the gating compliance and a calcium-dependent feedback that supplies energy to overcome damping effects on the hair bundle (Crawford et al., 1991; Markin & Hudspeth, 1995a, 1995b; Martin & Hudspeth, 1999; Martin et al., 2000; Ricci et al., 1998; Wu et al., 1999). What the transfer function is between hair bundle movements and basilar membrane or tectorial membrane movements remains unclear. Additional questions include: what are the maximal forces that can be exerted by the hair bundle, and what component of the tectorial membrane stiffness do the hair bundles contribute? One estimate suggests hair bundles dominate the mechanical properties of the tectorial membrane (Benser, Issa, & Hudspeth, 1993).

Even if fast adaptation and the corresponding hair bundle movements only make a small contribution to the active process, it is possible that the mechanical tuning mechanism is important for tuning of the free-standing inner hair cell bundles. Transducer properties of inner hair cells remains unknown. Mechanical tuning may be an important filtering mechanism for these hair cells.

Tonotopic variations have been found in a multitude of hair cell properties. From morphological differences like number and size of stereocilia to innervation (Hackney et al., 1993) differences like the variation in number of afferent synapses, (Sneary, 1988) tonotopic differences exist. Evidence demonstrates differences in the number and types of calcium and potassium channels present (Art & Fettiplace, 1987; Jones, Gray-Keller, Art, & Fettiplace, 1999; Ricci, Gray-Keller, et al., 2000; Wu, Art, Goodman, & Fettiplace, 1995; Wu & Fettiplace, 1996; Wu, Tucker, & Fettiplace, 1996), differences in calcium buffer concentrations (Ricci et al., 1998; Ricci, Gray-Keller, et al., 2000) as well as differences in the number of transducer channels and the rates of transducer adaptation, (Ricci & Fettiplace, 1997; Ricci et al., 1998). What are the developmental cues for this complex differentiating pattern of diverse properties? At what point in development is the tonotopic map layed out? What other properties vary? Can these developmental cues be restored in order to generate mature hair cells with all of the tonotopic variations present? How plastic is this tonotopic map?

What underlies the tonotopic variations in transducer properties? Certainly some evidence exists that summation is important (Ricci et al., 1998), but summation of what? Is the force generated by each channel summed, or is summation simply a reflection of the peak calcium levels changing? It is possible that the transducer channels are intrinsically different, much like the Bk potassium channels (Jones et al., 1999; Oberholtzer, 1999; Ramanathan, Michael, Jiang, Heil, & Fuchs, 1999; Ricci, Gray-Keller, et al., 2000). Intrinsic differences in calcium sensitivity or kinetics might underlie some of the measured differences in adaptation. Or does summation, an increase in the number of transducer channels per stereocilia, completely explain the tonotopic differences?

Where are the transducer channels located? As previously demonstrated, clear identification of the channel location is critical for evaluation of possible mechanisms involved in adaptation as well as for the identification of the proteins involved in the transduction process. Presently, data are at odds; however, most theories suggest the channels are at either or both ends of the tip-link. The tip-link may simply be a structural element used to keep the stereocilia in close approximation. If channels are not located at either ends of the tip-links, then to what does the myosin immunocytochemistry correspond? Myosins play many crucial roles in cell physiology, only one of which may be to control classical adaptation. So interpretation of function based on localization is tenuous. In fact, the finding of a fast component of adaptation means it is possible that classical adaptation mechanisms are located farther from the channel than previously suspected. A mechanism located at the base of the stereocilia regulating either the passive stiffness of the stereocilia or the resting position of the hair bundle would be a potent means of regulating the sensitivity of the hair bundle. A location closer to the base of the stereocilia would also explain the different displacement sensitivity of the two components of transducer adaptation. As more information is obtained about the complexities of signal processing in the inner ear, more questions arise. It is hoped the increase in our basic knowledge of the functioning of the inner ear will serve as a bridge to future clinically relevant applications, opening new and exciting avenues of intervention.

Acknowledgments: My thanks to Robert Fettiplace and Andrew Crawford who have been involved in the majority of these experiments. This work was supported by a Deafness Research Foundation Grant and by RO1DC03896 from National Institute of Deafness and other Communication Disorders (NIDCD).

REFERENCES

Art, J. J., & Fettiplace, R. (1987). Variation of membrane properties in hair cells isolated from the turtle cochlea. *The Journal of Physiology (London), 385,* 207–242.

Assad, J. A., & Corey, D. P. (1992). An active motor model for adaptation by vertebrate hair cells. *Journal of Neuroscience, 12,* 3291–3309.

Assad, J. A., Hacohen, N., & Corey, D. P. (1989). Voltage dependence of adaptation and active bundle movement in bullfrog saccular hair cells. *Proceedings of the National Academy of Sciences, USA, 86,* 2918–2922.

Benser, M. E., Issa, N. P., & Hudspeth, A. J. (1993). Hair-bundle stiffness dominates the elastic reactance to otolithic-membrane shear. *Hearing Research, 68,* 243–252.

Benser, M. E., Marquis, R. E., & Hudspeth, A. J. (1996). Rapid, active hair bundle movements in hair cells from the bullfrog's sacculus. *Journal of Neuroscience, 16,* 5629–5643.

Bosher, S. K., & Warren, R. L. (1978). Very low calcium content of cochlear endolymph, an extracellular fluid. *Nature, 273,* 377–378.

Brown, A. M., McDowell, B., & Forge, A. (1989). Acoustic distortion products can be used to monitor the effects of chronic gentamicin treatment. *Hearing Research, 42,* 143–156.

Burlacu, S., Tap, W. D., Lumpkin, E. A., & Hudspeth, A. J. (1997). ATPase activity of myosin in hair bundles of the bullfrog's sacculus. *Biophysical Journal, 72,* 263–271.

Corey, D. P., & Hudspeth, A. J. (1979). Response latency of vertebrate hair cells. *Biophysical Journal, 26,* 499–506.

Crawford, A. C., Evans, M. G., & Fettiplace, R. (1989). Activation and adaptation of transducer currents in turtle hair cells. *The Journal of Physiology (London), 419,* 405–434.

Crawford, A. C., Evans, M. G., & Fettiplace, R. (1991). The actions of calcium on the mechano-electrical transducer current of turtle hair cells. *The Journal of Physiology (London), 434,* 369–398.

Crawford, A. C., & Fettiplace, R. (1980). The frequency selectivity of auditory nerve fibres and hair cells in the cochlea of the turtle. *The Journal of Physiology (London), 306,* 79–125.

Crawford, A. C., & Fettiplace, R. (1985). The mechanical properties of ciliary bundles of turtle cochlear hair cells. *The Journal of Physiology (London), 364,* 359–379.

Denk, W., Holt, J. R., Shepherd, G. M., & Corey, D. P. (1995). Calcium imaging of single stereocilia in hair cells: localization of transduction channels at both ends of tip links. *Neuron, 15,* 1311–1321.

Eatock, R. A., Corey, D. P., & Hudspeth, A. J. (1987). Adaptation of mechano-electrical transduction in hair cells of the bullfrog's sacculus. *Journal of Neuroscience, 7,* 2821–2836.

Fettiplace, R., & Fuchs, P. A. (1999). Mechanisms of hair cell tuning. *Annual Review of Physiology, 61,* 809–834.

Furness, D. N., Hackney, C. M., & Benos, D. J. (1996). The binding site on cochlear stereocilia for antisera raised against renal Na+ channels is blocked by amiloride and dihydrostreptomycin. *Hearing Research, 93,* 136–146.

Garcia, J. A., Yee, A. G., Gillespie, P. G., & Corey, D. P. (1998). Localization of myosin-Ibeta near both ends of tip links in frog saccular hair cells. *Journal of Neuroscience, 18,* 8637–8647.

Geleoc, G. S., Lennan, G. W., Richardson, G. P., & Kros, C. J. (1997). A quantitative comparison of mechanoelectrical transduction in vestibular and auditory hair cells of neonatal mice. *Proceedings of the Royal Society of London, Series B, Biological Sciences, 264,* 611–621.

Gillespie, P. G. (1997). Multiple myosin motors and mechanoelectrical transduction by hair cells. *The Biological Bulletin, 192,* 186–190.

Gillespie, P. G., & Corey, D. P. (1997). Myosin and adaptation by hair cells. *Neuron, 19,* 955–958.

Gillespie, P. G., & Hudspeth, A. J. (1993). Adenine nucleoside diphosphates block adaptation of mechanoelectrical transduction in hair cells. *Proceedings of the National Academy of Sciences, USA, 90,* 2710–2714.

Gillespie, P. G., Wagner, M. C., & Hudspeth, A. J. (1993). Identification of a 120 kd hair-bundle myosin located near stereociliary tips. *Neuron, 11,* 581–594.

Hackney, C. M., Fettiplace, R., & Furness, D. N. (1993). The functional morphology of stereociliary bundles on turtle cochlear hair cells. *Hearing Research, 69,* 163–175.

Hackney, C. M., Furness, D. N., Benos, D. J., Woodley, J. F., & Barratt, J. (1992). Putative immunolocalization of the mechanoelectrical transduction channels in mammalian cochlear hair cells. *Proceedings of the Royal Society of London, Series B, Biological Sciences, 248,* 215–221.

Hacohen, N., Assad, J. A., Smith, W. J., & Corey, D. P. (1989). Regulation of tension on hair-cell transduction channels: Displacement and calcium dependence. *Journal of Neuroscience, 9,* 3988–3997.

Holt, J. R., Corey, D. P., & Eatock, R. A. (1997). Mechanoelectrical transduction and adaptation in hair cells of the mouse utricle, a low-frequency vestibular organ. *Journal of Neuroscience, 17,* 8739–8748.

Howard, J., & Ashmore, J. F. (1986). Stiffness of sensory hair bundles in the sacculus of the frog. *Hearing Research, 23,* 93–104.

Howard, J., & Hudspeth, A. J. (1987). Mechanical relaxation of the hair bundle mediates adaptation in mechanoelectrical transduction by the bullfrog's saccular hair cell. *Proceedings of the National Academy of Sciences, USA, 84,* 3064–3068.

Howard, J., & Hudspeth, A. J. (1988). Compliance of the hair bundle associated with gating of mechanoelectrical transduction channels in the bullfrog's saccular hair cell. *Neuron, 1,* 189–199.

Hudspeth, A. J. (1982). Extracellular current flow and the site of transduction by vertebrate hair cells. *Journal of Neuroscience, 2,* 1–10.

Hudspeth, A. J., & Corey, D. P. (1977). Sensitivity, polarity, and conductance change in the response of vertebrate hair cells to controlled mechanical stimuli. *Proceedings of the National Academy of Sciences, USA, 74,* 2407–2411.

Jaramillo, F., & Hudspeth, A. J. (1991). Localization of the hair cell's transduction channels at the hair bundle's top by iontophoretic application of a channel blocker. *Neuron, 7,* 409–420.

Jones, E. M., Gray-Keller, M., Art, J. J., & Fettiplace, R. (1999). The functional role of alternative splicing of Ca(2+)-activated K+ channels in auditory hair cells. *Annals of the New York Academy of Sciences, 868,* 379–385.

Jorgensen, F., & Kroese, A. B. (1994). Ionic selectivity of the mechano-electrical transduction channels in the hair cells of the frog sacculus. *Acta Physiologica Scandinavia, 151,* 7–16.

Jorgensen, F., & Kroese, A. B. (1995). Ca selectivity of the transduction channels in the hair cells of the frog sacculus. *Acta Physiologica Scandinavia, 155,* 363–376.

Jorgensen, F., & Ohmori, H. (1988). Amiloride blocks the mechano-electrical transduction channel of hair cells of the chick. *The Journal of Physiology (London), 403,* 577–588.

Koppl, C., & Manley, G. A. (1993). Spontaneous otoacoustic emissions in the bobtail lizard. I: General characteristics. *Hearing Research, 71,* 157–169.

Kros, C. J., Rusch, A., & Richardson, G. P. (1992). Mechano-electrical transducer currents in hair cells of the cultured neonatal mouse cochlea. *Proceedings of the Royal Society of London, Series B, Biological Sciences, 249,* 185–193.

Kros, J. M. (1995). Oligodendrogliomas: Clinicopathological correlations. *Journal of Neuro-oncology, 24(1),* 29–31.

Lumpkin, E. A., & Hudspeth, A. J. (1995). Detection of Ca2+ entry through mechanosensitive channels localizes the site of mechanoelectrical transduction in hair cells. *Proceedings of the National Academy of Sciences, USA, 92,* 10297–10301.

Lumpkin, E. A., Marquis, R. E., & Hudspeth, A. J. (1997). The selectivity of the hair cell's mechanoelectrical-transduction channel promotes Ca2+ flux at low Ca2+ concentrations. *Proceedings of the National Academy of Sciences, USA, 94*, 10997–11002.

Markin, V. S., & Hudspeth, A. J. (1995a). Gating-spring models of mechano-electrical transduction by hair cells of the internal ear. *Annual Review of Biophysics and Biomolecular Structure, 24*, 59–83.

Markin, V. S., & Hudspeth, A. J. (1995b). Modeling the active process of the cochlea: Phase relations, amplification, and spontaneous oscillation. *Biophysical Journal, 69*, 138–147.

Marquis, R. E., & Hudspeth, A. J. (1997). Effects of extracellular Ca2+ concentration on hair-bundle stiffness and gating-spring integrity in hair cells. *Proceedings of the National Academy of Sciences, USA, 94*, 11923–11928.

Martin, P., & Hudspeth, A. J. (1999). Active hair-bundle movements can amplify a hair cell's response to oscillatory mechanical stimuli. *Proceedings of the National Academy of Sciences, USA, 96*, 14306–14311.

Martin, P., Mehta, A. D., & Hudspeth, A. J. (2000). Negative hair-bundle stiffness betrays a mechanism for mechanical amplification by the hair cell [In Process Citation]. *Proceedings of the National Academy of Sciences, USA, 97*, 12026–12031.

Metcalf, A. B., Chelliah, Y., & Hudspeth, A. J. (1994). Molecular cloning of a myosin I beta isozyme that may mediate adaptation by hair cells of the bullfrog's internal ear. *Proceedings of the National Academy of Sciences, USA, 91*, 11821–11825.

Nobili, R., Mammano, F., & Ashmore, J. (1998). How well do we understand the cochlea? *Trends in Neuroscience, 21*, 159–167.

Oberholtzer, J. C. (1999). Frequency tuning of cochlear hair cells by differential splicing of BK channel transcripts [editorial; comment]. *The Journal of Physiology (London), 518*, 629.

Ohmori, H. (1985). Mechano-electrical transduction currents in isolated vestibular hair cells of the chick. *The Journal of Physiology (London), 359*, 189–217.

Ohmori, H. (1988). Mechanical stimulation and Fura-2 fluorescence in the hair bundle of dissociated hair cells of the chick. *The Journal of Physiology (London), 399*, 115–137.

Pickles, J. O., Brix, J., Comis, S. D., Gleich, O., Koppl, C., Manley, G. A., & Osborne, M. P. (1989). The organization of tip links and stereocilia on hair cells of bird and lizard basilar papillae. *Hearing Research, 41*, 31–41.

Probst, R., Lonsbury-Martin, B. L., & Martin, G. K. (1991). A review of otoacoustic emissions. *The Journal of the Acoustical Society of America, 89*, 2027–2067.

Ramanathan, K., Michael, T. H., Jiang, G. J., Hiel, H., & Fuchs, P. A. (1999). A molecular mechanism for electrical tuning of cochlear hair cells. *Science, 283*, 215–217.

Ricci, A. J., Crawford, A. C., & Fettiplace, R. (2000a). Active hair bundle motion linked to fast transducer adaptation in auditory hair cells [In Process Citation]. *Journal of Neuroscience, 20*, 7131–7142.

Ricci, A. J., & Fettiplace, R. (1997). The effects of calcium buffering and cyclic AMP on mechano-electrical transduction in turtle auditory hair cells. *The Journal of Physiology (London), 501,* 111–124.

Ricci, A. J., & Fettiplace, R. (1998). Calcium permeation of the turtle hair cell mechanotransducer channel and its relation to the composition of endolymph [published erratum appears in *The Journal of Physiology (London)* (1998) 507(Pt. 3), 939]. *The Journal of Physiology (London), 506,* 159–173.

Ricci, A. J., Gray-Keller, M., & Fettiplace, R. (2000b). Tonotopic variations of calcium signalling in turtle auditory hair cells. *The Journal of Physiology (London), 524*(Pt. 2), 423–436.

Ricci, A. J., Wu, Y. C., & Fettiplace, R. (1998). The endogenous calcium buffer and the time course of transducer adaptation in auditory hair cells. *Journal of Neuroscience, 18,* 8261–8277.

Roberts, W. M., Howard, J., & Hudspeth, A. J. (1988). Hair cells: Transduction, tuning, and transmission in the inner ear. *Annual Review of Cell Biology, 4,* 63–92.

Rusch, A., Kros, C. J., & Richardson, G. P. (1994). Block by amiloride and its derivatives of mechano-electrical transduction in outer hair cells of mouse cochlear cultures. *The Journal of Physiology (London), 474,* 75–86.

Russell, I. J., Richardson, G. P., & Kossl, M. (1989). The responses of cochlear hair cells to tonic displacements of the sensory hair bundle. *Hearing Research, 43,* 55–69.

Shepherd, G. M., & Corey, D. P. (1994). The extent of adaptation in bullfrog saccular hair cells. *Journal of Neuroscience, 14,* 6217–6229.

Shotwell, S. L., Jacobs, R., & Hudspeth, A. J. (1981). Directional sensitivity of individual vertebrate hair cells to controlled deflection of their hair bundles. *Annals of the New York Academy of Sciences, 374,* 1–10.

Sneary, M. G. (1988). Auditory receptor of the red-eared turtle: II. Afferent and efferent synapses and innervation patterns. *The Journal of Comparative Neurology, 276,* 588–606.

Stewart, C. E., & Hudspeth, A. J. (2000). Effects of salicylates and aminoglycosides on spontaneous otoacoustic emissions in the Tokay gecko. *Proceedings of the National Academy of Sciences, USA, 97,* 454–459.

Steyger, P. S., Gillespie, P. G., & Baird, R. A. (1998). Myosin Ibeta is located at tip link anchors in vestibular hair bundles. *Journal of Neuroscience, 18,* 4603–4615.

Tilney, L. G., & DeRosier, D. J. (1986). Actin filaments, stereocilia, and hair cells of the bird cochlea. IV. How the actin filaments become organized in developing stereocilia and in the cuticular plate. *Developmental Biology, 116,* 119–129.

Tilney, L. G., Derosier, D. J., & Mulroy, M. J. (1980). The organization of actin filaments in the stereocilia of cochlear hair cells. *The Journal of Cell Biology, 86,* 244–259.

Tilney, L. G., Egelman, E. H., DeRosier, D. J., & Saunder, J. C. (1983). Actin filaments, stereocilia, and hair cells of the bird cochlea. II. Packing of actin filaments in the stereocilia and in the cuticular plate and what happens to the organization when the stereocilia are bent. *The Journal of Cell Biology, 96,* 822–834.

Tilney, L. G., & Saunders, J. C. (1983). Actin filaments, stereocilia, and hair cells of the bird cochlea. I. Length, number, width, and distribution of stereocilia of each hair cell are related to the position of the hair cell on the cochlea. *The Journal of Cell Biology, 96,* 807–821.

Tilney, L. G., Tilney, M. S., Saunders, J. S., & DeRosier, D. J. (1986). Actin filaments, stereocilia, and hair cells of the bird cochlea. III. The development and differentiation of hair cells and stereocilia. *Developmental Biology, 116,* 100–118.

van Netten, S. M., & Kros, C. J. (2000). Gating energies and forces of the mammalian hair cell transducer channel and related hair bundle mechanics [In Process Citation]. *Proceedings of the Royal Society of London, Series B, Biological Sciences, 267,* 1915–1923.

Wolfrum, U., Liu, X., Schmitt, A., Udovichenko, I. P., & Williams, D. S. (1998). Myosin VIIa as a common component of cilia and microvilli. *Cell Motility and the Cytoskeleton, 40,* 261–271.

Wu, Y. C., Art, J. J., Goodman, M. B., & Fettiplace, R. (1995). A kinetic description of the calcium-activated potassium channel and its application to electrical tuning of hair cells. *Progress in Biophysics and Molecular Biology, 63,* 131–158.

Wu, Y. C., & Fettiplace, R. (1996). A developmental model for generating frequency maps in the reptilian and avian cochleas. *Biophysical Journal, 70,* 2557–2570.

Wu, Y. C., Ricci, A. J., & Fettiplace, R. (1999). Two components of transducer adaptation in auditory hair cells. *Journal of Neurophysiology, 82,* 2171–2181.

Wu, Y. C., Tucker, T., & Fettiplace, R. (1996). A theoretical study of calcium microdomains in turtle hair cells. *Biophysical Journal, 71,* 2256–2275.

Yamoah, E. N., & Gillespie, P. G. (1996). Phosphate analogs block adaptation in hair cells by inhibiting adaptation-motor force production. *Neuron, 17,* 523–533.

Modulation of the Resting Potassium Current in Type I Vestibular Hair Cells by cGMP

K. J. Rennie, PhD
Department of Otolaryngology
University of Texas Medical Branch
Galveston, Texas

INTRODUCTION

Type I hair cells are found in the vestibular epithelia of amniotes and are innervated by an afferent nerve calyx (Wersäll, 1956). Efferent fibers make synaptic contact with the outer face of the calyx, whereas the inner face of the calyx almost completely surrounds the basolateral membrane of the type I hair cell. Type I hair cells differ morphologically and electrophysiologically from type II hair cells. Recordings in whole cell patch clamp have shown that a large delayed rectifier K^+ current (I_{KI} or I_{KL}) is active at unusually negative membrane potentials in type I vestibular hair cells and is absent from type II hair cells (Correia & Lang, 1990; Rennie & Correia, 1994; Rüsch & Eatock, 1996). Consequently, type I hair cells have a low input resistance and are predicted to show smaller membrane potential excursions than type II hair cells in response to deflections of their stereocilia (Rennie & Correia, 1994). Furthermore, the type I hair cell K^+ conductance has recently been shown to be modulated through a nitric oxide (NO)/cyclic guanosine monophosphate (cGMP) signaling pathway, whereby NO donors or cGMP decrease the size of the conductance (Behrend, Schwark, Kunhiro, & Strupp, 1997; Chen & Eatock, 2000). NO is thought to stimulate cGMP production through the activation of soluble guanylate cyclase, which is reported to be present in the vestibular neuroepithelium (Hess et al., 1998). The mechanism whereby cGMP regulates the K^+ current is not known, but since the effect is observed in whole cell recordings and not in excised patches, it is thought not to involve a direct effect of cGMP on the channel (Behrend et al., 1997). Two alternative pathways by which cGMP could inhibit the resting K^+ conductance in isolated type I vestibular hair cells are investigated here.

METHODS

Cell Preparation

Hair cells were nonenzymatically dissociated from the semicircular canals and utricles of Mongolian gerbils as described previously (Rennie & Correia, 2000). Procedures were carried out in accordance with the American Physiological Society guidelines and were approved by The University of Texas Medical Branch Animal Care and Use Committee. Gerbils were injected with Nembutal (50 mg/kg ip) and ketamine (40 mg/kg im), and the vestibular end organs were removed under deep anesthesia. End organs were placed in a chilled solution containing (in mM): NaCl (135), KCl (5), $MgCl_2$ (10), $CaCl_2$ (0.02), NaH_2PO_4 (2), Na_2HPO_4 (8) and D-glucose (3), pH 7.4 with NaOH and osmolality 305 mmol/kg. Animals were decapitated immediately following end organ removal. Epithelia were incubated for 32 minutes at 37°C and then transferred to a solution of Leibovitz's L-15 medium (Life Technologies) containing bovine albumin (1 mg/ml) for at least 50 minutes at room temperature (20–22°C). Individual epithelia were then placed in standard L-15 medium in the recording chamber, and the epithelial surface was stroked with a probe to dislodge hair cells. Cells were viewed on a Nikon inverted microscope and identified by morphological characteristics (Ricci, Rennie, Cochran, Kevetter, & Correia, 1997).

Electrophysiological Recording and Solutions

Conventional whole cell tight-seal patch clamp experiments were carried out at room temperature. Electrodes were pulled on a Sutter Instruments microelectrode puller (P-87) from capillary tubing (Warner Instrument Corp. PG165T), coated with silicone elastomer (Sylgard, Dow Corning), and the tips were viewed and heat-polished on a microforge (Narashige MF 83). The standard electrode solution was (in mM): KF (110), KCl (15), KOH (27), NaCl (1), HEPES (10), D-glucose (3), $MgCl_2$ (1.8) and EGTA (10), pH 7.4.

Current recordings from dissociated hair cells were made with an Axopatch-1C or 1D patch amplifier connected to an IBM equivalent personal computer through an AD converter (CED 1401, Cambridge Electronic Design). Stimuli were generated and data acquired using CED Patch and Voltage Clamp software (V 6). Signals were low-pass filtered online at 2-5 kHz. Cell capacitance had a mean value of 2.7 ± 0.8 pF (n = 16), and capacitance transients were cancelled at the start of the recording using the compensation circuitry of the amplifiers. Series resistance was 4.2 ± 2.6 MΩ (n = 16) and was compensated up to 80%.

The extracellular superfusion solution was L-15. Chemicals were obtained from Biomol (Plymouth Meeting, PA) or Sigma (St. Louis, MO). Drugs were applied via a series of flow pipes placed close to the cell under study.

Data Analysis

Analyses were performed and figures generated using Sigmaplot (Jandel Scientific). Values presented are means ± SD.

RESULTS

Figure 4–1A shows typical currents recorded from an isolated gerbil type I hair cell. In control conditions, a large instantaneous component to the current is evident in response to hyperpolarizing and depolarizing steps from the holding potential of −70 mV. The decline of the current following a hyperpolarizing step to −90 mV represents deactivation of the current, which is active at the holding potential. This current has previously been identified as a low-voltage activated delayed rectifier current and gives rise to the low input resistance of type I hair cells (Rennie & Correia, 1994; Rüsch & Eatock, 1996). In the right panel of Figure 4–1A, currents in the same cell following extracellular perfusion of the membrane-permeant form of cGMP, 8-bromoadenosine 3′, 5′-cyclic monophosphate (8-Br-cGMP, 1 mM) are shown.

The effect of 8-Br-cGMP was to inhibit the resting conductance and slow the activation kinetics of the outward current. Since the major effect was on the instantaneous component, a voltage ramp protocol was also used to assess the action of cGMP (Figure 4–1B). Control current and current following application of 1 mM 8-Br-cGMP are shown. In the presence of 8-Br-cGMP, currents were reduced to

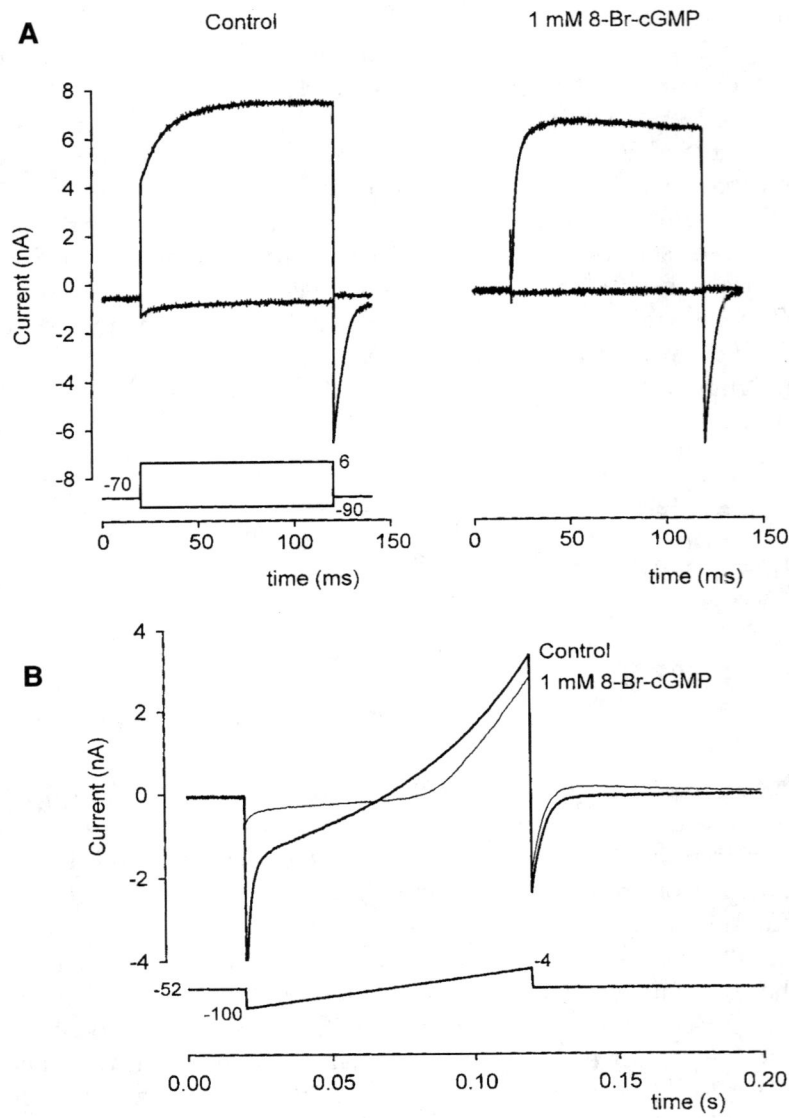

Figure 4–1. Inhibition of K$^+$ current in type I hair cells by cGMP. The membrane-permeant form of cGMP, 8-Br-cGMP, was applied to a type I hair cell under whole cell voltage-clamp. (**A**) Control currents (left) and currents in response to extracellular application of 1 mM 8-Br-cGMP (right) during voltage steps to a hyperpolarized (–90 mV) and depolarized (+6 mV) potential from a holding potential of –70 mV. (**B**) Reduction of instantaneous currents in the same cell in response to application of 8-Br-cGMP (thin trace) during a voltage ramp. Cell was held at –52 mV, and voltage ramps were applied between the potentials indicated (shown below).

53.5 ± 20.1% of control ($n = 11$). Although I_{KI} can show spontaneous shifts in its activation range over time (Rennie & Correia, 1994; Rüsch & Eatock, 1996), such shifts were ruled out in these experiments by monitoring currents for stability for several minutes prior to 8-Br-cGMP application. 8-Br-cGMP typically reduced currents within 30–60 sec from the start of application, and the effects of 8-Br-cGMP were often reversible (see Figure 4–2).

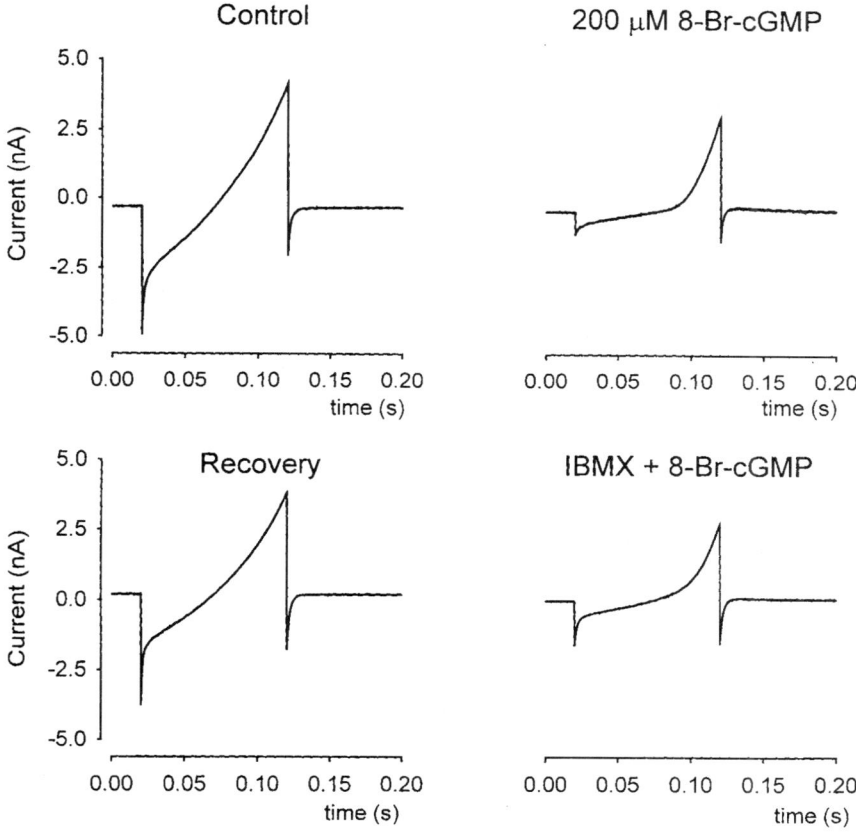

Figure 4–2. Effect of 3-isobutyl-1-methylxanthine (IBMX) on the response to cGMP. 8-Br-cGMP reduced the resting conductance in a type I hair cell (top right). Currents returned to near control values following return to normal extracellular solution (Recovery, bottom left). To test whether cGMP acts through a phosphodiesterase, 200 μM 8-Br-cGMP was subsequently applied to the cell in the presence of the nonspecific phosphodiesterase inhibitor IBMX. Application of 100 μM IBMX did not inhibit the response to 8-Br-cGMP. For the cell shown, each plot represents the average of 5 current responses obtained during voltage ramps applied from a holding potential of –70 mV.

IBMX DOES NOT INHIBIT THE RESPONSE TO cGMP

Cyclic GMP can mediate intracellular effects through cGMP-dependent phosphodiesterase, which can modulate levels of cAMP or cGMP (Lucas et al., 2000). IBMX (3-isobutyl-1-methylxanthine) is a nonspecific phosphodiesterase inhibitor, and to test whether cGMP exerts its effect on I_{KI} through phosphodiesterase, 200 µM 8-Br-cGMP was applied to cells in the presence of 100 µM IBMX. As shown in Figure 4–2, application of IBMX did not block the response to 8-Br-cGMP. Furthermore, IBMX had no effect on currents when applied alone (not shown). When applied together 8-Br-cGMP and IBMX reduced currents by 81.6 ± 12.2% ($n = 4$), suggesting that the inhibitory action of cGMP on I_{KI} is not mediated by a phosphodiesterase KT5823, the protein kinase G inhibitor, reduces the response to cGMP.

To investigate whether protein kinase G plays a role in the response of type I hair cells to cGMP KT5823, a specific inhibitor of protein kinase G was applied to cells together with 8-Br-cGMP. Figure 4–3 shows control current, current in the presence of 1 µM KT5823, and current in the presence of KT5823 and 200 µM 8-Br-cGMP. In the presence of KT5823 and 8-Br-cGMP, currents were 93.5 ± 5.9% of values in 1 µM KT5823 alone and were significantly different from responses to 8-Br-cGMP alone ($p < 0.05$, student's t-test) (Figure 4–4). The responses of type I hair cells to 8-Br-cGMP alone and 8-Br-cGMP applied in the presence of IBMX or KT5823 are summarized in Figure 4–4. Results indicate that cGMP acts through the stimulation of PKG to reduce I_{KI}.

DISCUSSION

This study shows that cGMP inhibits g_{KI}, the large resting K$^+$ conductance in gerbil type I vestibular hair cells. Previous results from type I hair cells isolated from rat semicircular canals showed that cGMP produced a rightwards shift of approximately 15 mV in the half-activation of I_{KI} and reduced channel open probability (Behrend et al., 1997). NO donors, such as sodium nitroprusside, also reduced the whole cell resting conductance in type I hair cells (Chen & Eatock, 2000). These previous observations demonstrated that a NO/cGMP modulatory pathway exists in type I hair cells. Application of cGMP or sodium nitroprusside to excised patches failed to inhibit the activity of I_{KI} channels in rat vestibular type I hair cells, ruling out a direct effect of

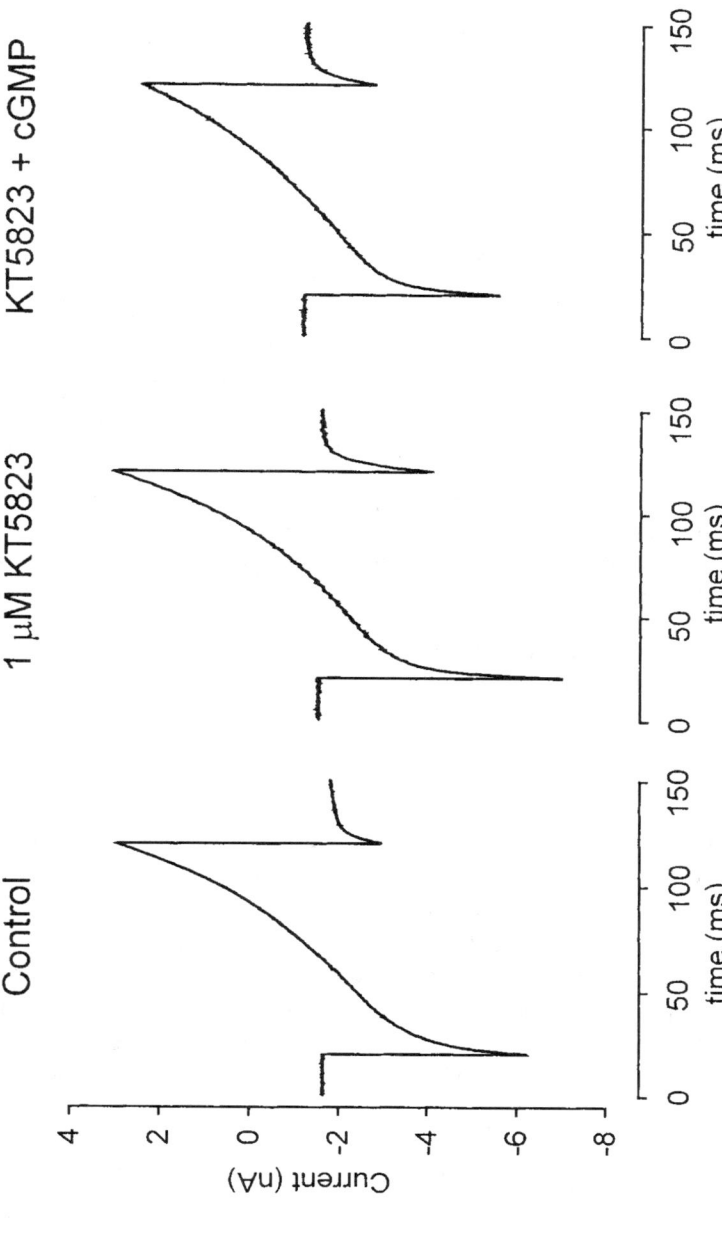

Figure 4-3. KT5823, an inhibitor of PKG, blocks the response to 8-Br-cGMP. Control current (left), current in the presence of 1 μM KT5823 (center) and current in the presence of KT5823 and 200 μM 8-Br-cGMP (right) are indicated. Each trace represents the average of 3–5 current responses obtained during voltage ramps applied from a holding potential of –70 mV.

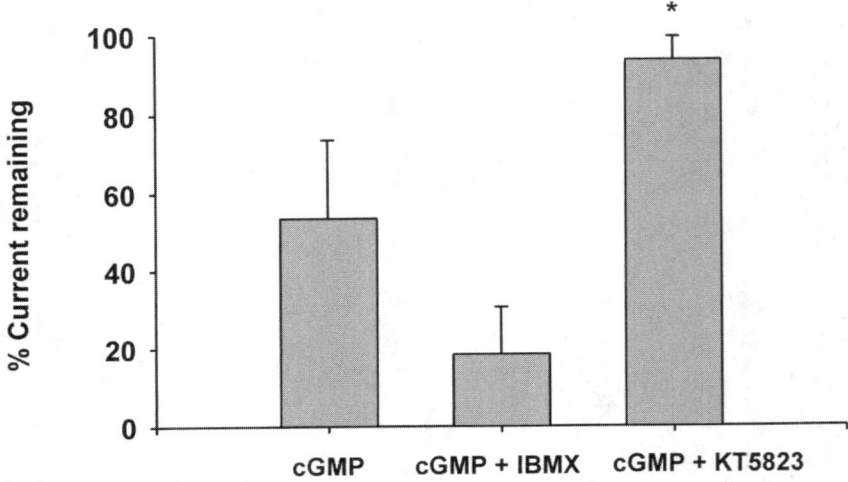

Figure 4–4. A summary of the effects of 8-Br-cGMP and inhibitors on type I hair cell currents. Current values were obtained from ramp protocols at –90 mV (holding potential –70 mV) and expressed as a percent of control values. 8-Br-cGMP (200 mM) reduces currents to near half control values 53.5 ± 20.1% ($n = 11$). In the presence of the phosphodiesterase inhibitor IBMX (200 µM), 8-Br-cGMP continued to elicit a large reduction in current amplitude ($n = 4$). When applied in the presence of the PKG inhibitor KT5823 (1 µM), responses to cGMP were greatly attenuated ($n = 3$) and were significantly different from responses to 8-Br-cGMP alone (unpaired t-test, $*p < 0.05$).

cGMP on the channel (Behrend et al., 1997; Chen & Eatock, 2000). Two alternative routes of action for cGMP are (a) through a phosphodiesterase or (b) through activation of protein kinase G. Results presented here suggest that the cGMP effect is not mediated through a phosphodiesterase, since application of the nonspecific phosphodiesterase inhibitor IBMX did not block the response to cGMP. In contrast, the PKG inhibitor, KT5823, at a concentration that selectively inhibits protein kinase G (Kase et al., 1987), markedly inhibited the response to cGMP. This indicates that cGMP decreases channel activity via activation of PKG.

The presence of I_{KI} confers a low input resistance on type I hair cells (Rennie & Correia, 1994; Rüsch & Eatock, 1996). Recent evidence suggests that KCNQ4 channels may contribute to this current and to $I_{K,n}$ in outer hair cells of the cochlea (Kubisch et al., 1999; Kharkovets et al., 2000; Marcotti & Kros, 1999; Rennie, Weng, & Correia, 2001). Although modulation of KCNQ channels by cGMP has not been described previously, other potassium channels are known to be influenced by cGMP. For example, a cGMP-activated K^+ channel is present in the cortical collecting duct of the rat kidney, and the NO/cGMP effect in this system also appears to be mediated by PKG (Wang, 2000). In addition, cGMP increases the activity of a calcium-activated K^+ channel in smooth muscle cells through PKG (Archer et al., 1994).

In the mammalian inner ear, A NO/cGMP/PKG pathway is reported to regulate intracellular calcium in Deiters' and Hensen's cells of the guinea pig cochlea (Matsunobu & Schacht, 2000). NO has also recently been implicated in cephalopod equilibrium receptor organ function. In the cuttlefish statocyst, a NO/cGMP pathway inhibits the resting activity of afferent fibers, whereas a NO/cAMP pathway increases afferent activity (Tu & Budelmann, 2000). In the mammalian vestibular system, efferent stimulation produces a predominantly excitatory effect on afferent firing pattern (Goldberg & Fernandez, 1980). The following scheme suggests a mechanism whereby NO acting on type I hair cells could produce the excitatory response seen in vestibular primary afferents. As a result of the high input conductance of type I hair cells, only small changes in receptor potential amplitude will occur in response to hair bundle stimulation. Activation of a NO/cGMP/PKG cascade would serve to reduce I_{KI}, thereby increasing the input resistance and enhancing the sensitivity of type I hair cells to mechanotransduction currents. A possible route for this could be through activation of the efferent fibers, which do not contact type I hair cells directly, but synapse onto the outer face of the calyx fibers innervating type I hair cells. Nitric oxide synthase I is reported to be present in vestibular efferent fibers and a minority of hair cells (Lysakowski & Singer, 2000). Following depolarization and calcium influx through voltage-dependent calcium channels, nitric oxide produced by both efferent fibers and hair cells could diffuse through the epithelium and activate the NO/cGMP/PKG pathway leading to a reduction in I_{KI} and an enhanced type I hair cell response. This could then lead to an increase in firing in those afferents innervating type I hair cells.

Acknowledgment: Supported by National Institute of Deafness and other Communication Disorders (NIDCD) grant DC03287. I thank Manning J. Correia, PhD, for the loan of equipment.

REFERENCES

Archer, S. L., Huang, J. M., Hampl, V., Nelson, D. P., Schultz, P. J., & Weir, E. K. (1994). Nitric oxide and cGMP cause vasorelaxation by activation of a charybdotoxin-sensitive K channel by cGMP-dependent protein kinase. *Proceedings of the National Academy of Sciences, USA, 91*, 7583–7587.

Behrend, O., Schwark, C., Kunihiro, T., & Strupp, M. (1997). Cyclic GMP inhibits and shifts the activation curve of the delayed-rectifier (I[K1]) of type I mammalian vestibular hair cells. *Neuroreport, 8*, 2687–2690.

Chen, J. W. Y., & Eatock, R. A. (2000). Major potassium conductance in type I hair cells from rat semicircular canals: Characterization and modulation by nitric oxide. *Journal of Neurophysiology, 84*, 139–151.

Correia, M. J., & Lang, D. G. (1990). An electrophysiological comparison of solitary type I and type II vestibular hair cells. *Neuroscience Letters, 116*, 106–111.

Goldberg, J. M., & Fernandez, C. (1980). Efferent vestibular system in the squirrel monkey: anatomical location and influence on afferent activity. *Journal of Neurophysiology, 43*, 986–1025.

Hess, A., Bloch, W., Su, J., Stennert, E., Addicks, K., & Michel, O. (1998). Localisation of the nitric oxide (NO)/cGMP-pathway in the vestibular system of guinea pigs. *Neuroscience Letters, 251*, 185–188.

Kase, H., Iwahashi, K., Nakanishi, S., Matsuda, Y., Yamada, K., Takahashi, M., Murakata, C., Sato, A., & Kaneko, M. (1987). K-252 compounds, novel and potent inhibitors of protein kinase C and cyclic nucleotide-dependent protein kinases. *Biochemical and Biophysical Research Communications, 142*, 436–440.

Kharkovets, T., Hardelin J.- P., Safieddine, S., Schweizer, M., El-Amraoui, A., Petit, C., & Jentsch, T. J. (2000). KCNQ4, a K+ channel mutated in a form of dominant deafness, is expressed in the inner ear and the central auditory pathway. *Proceedings of the National Academy of Sciences, USA, 97*, 4333–4338.

Kubisch, C., Schroeder, B. C., Friedrich, T., Lutjohann, B., El-Amraoui, A., Marline, S., Petit, C., & Jentsch, T. J. (1999). KCNQ4, a novel potassium channel expressed in sensory outer hair cells, is mutated in dominant deafness. *Cell, 94*, 437–446.

Lysakowski, A., & Singer, M. (2000). Nitric oxide synthase localized in a subpopulation of vestibular efferents with NADPH diaphorase histochemistry and nitric oxide synthase immunohistochemistry. *The Journal of Comparative Neurology, 427*, 508–521.

Marcotti, W., & Kros, C. J. (2000). Developmental expression of the potassium current IK,n contributes to maturation of mouse outer hair cells. *The Journal of Physiology, 520*, 653–660.

Matsunobu, T., & Schacht, J. (2000). Nitric oxide/cyclic GMP pathway attenuates ATP-evoked intracellular calcium increase in supporting cells of the guinea pig cochlea. *The Journal of Comparative Neurology, 423*, 452–461.

Rennie, K. J., & Correia, M. J. (1994). Potassium currents in mammalian and avian isolated type I semicircular canal hair cells. *Journal of Neurophysiology, 71,* 317–329.

Rennie, K. J., & Correia, M. J. (2000). Effects of cationic substitutions on delayed rectifier current in type I vestibular hair cells. *The Journal of Membrane Biology, 173,* 139–148.

Rennie, K. J., Weng, T. X., & Correia, M. J. (2001). Effects of KCNQ channel blockers on K(+) currents in vestibular hair cells. *American Journal of Physiology. Cell Physiology, 280,* 473–480.

Ricci, A. J., Rennie, K. J., Cochran S. L., Kevetter G. A., & Correia, M. J. (1997). Vestibular type I and type II hair cells. 1: Morphometric identification in the pigeon and gerbil. *Journal of Vestibular Research: Equilibrium & Orientation, 7,* 393–406.

Rüsch, A., & Eatock, R. A. (1996). A delayed rectifier conductance in type I hair cells of the mouse utricle. *Journal of Neurophysiology, 76,* 995–1004.

Tu, Y., & Budelmann, B. U. (2000). Effects of nitric oxide donors on the afferent resting activity in the cephalopod statocyst. *Brain Research, 865,* 211–220.

Wang, W. H. (2000). The cGMP-dependent protein kinase stimulates the basolateral 18-pS K channel of the rat CCD. *American Journal of Physiology. Cell Physiology, 278,* C1212–1217.

Wersäll, J. (1956). Studies on the structure and innervation of the sensory epithelium of the cristae ampullares in the guinea pig. *Acta Oto-laryngologica Supplememtum (Stockholm), 126,* 1–85.

Electrical and ATP Induced Movements of the Phalangeal Processes of Isolated Cochlear Deiters' Cells

Richard P. Bobbin, PhD
Julie Campbell, BS
Suzanne Lousteau
Manisha Mandhare, BS
Kresge Hearing Research Laboratory of the South
Department of Otorhinolaryngology and Biocommunication
Louisiana State University Health Sciences Center
New Orleans, Louisiana

INTRODUCTION

Currently, the role of extracellular adenosine triphosphate (ATP) at receptors on the cells of the cochlea is speculative (see reviews: Bobbin, 1996, 1997; Bobbin Chen, Nenov, & Skellett, 1998; Bobbin et al., 2000; Bobbin, LeBlanc, Mandhare, & Parker, 2001). There are receptors that are activated by extracellular ATP on cell surfaces exposed to endolymph and on cell surfaces exposed to perilymph (Housley, 1997; Housley et al., 1999; Parker, Larroque, Campbell, Bobbin, & Deininger, 1998; Xiang, Bo, & Burnstock, 1999). Undoubtedly, the ATP receptors exposed to endolymph are involved in fluid and ion movement across cells lining the scala media (e.g., Munoz, Kendrick, Rassam, & Thorne, 2001). Our laboratory has focused on the roles of ATP receptors exposed to perilymph (Bobbin & Thompson, 1978; Bobbin et al., 1998; Bobbin et al., 2000; Chen, Skellett, Fallon, & Bobbin, 1998; Skellett,

91

Chen, Fallon, Nenov, & Bobbin, 1997). One reason for this focus is our ability to place chemicals into the perilymph compartment where they have ready access to receptors on cell surfaces bathed by perilymph (e.g., Deiters' cells, hair cells, nerve cell terminals). When placed in perilymph, most ionized, hydrophillic chemicals such as ATP are thought to be prevented from penetration into endolymph by cellular barriers. Thus, chemicals placed in the perilymph compartment are in the unique position to selectively affect the receptors on cells in the organ of Corti exposed to perilymph separate from possible effects of the chemicals on receptors exposed to endolymph.

When placed into perilymph, chemicals that activate and block ATP receptors have dramatic effects on the mechanical motion of the cochlear partition and on the function of the organ of Corti as monitored by distortion product otoacoustic emissions (DPOAEs). The ATP receptor agonist, ATP-γ-S, decreases the magnitude of the cubic DPOAEs while simultaneously increasing the magnitude of the quadratic DPOAEs (Bobbin et al., 2000; Kujawa, Erostegui, Fallon, Crist, & Bobbin, 1994). Pyridoxal-phosphate-6-azophenyl-2',4'-disulphonic acid (PPADS), an ATP antagonist, has the opposite effect of ATP-γ-S. PPADS reduces the quadratic DPOAEs about 12 dB at 60 dB primary levels (Chen et al., 1998) and increases the cubic DPOAEs (Bobbin et al., 2000). Based on this pharmacological data, it seems that the magnitude of the cubic and quadratic DPOAEs may be a reflection of a modulatory role of extracellular ATP on cochlear mechanics via receptors exposed to perilymph. To date, these effects of ATP agonists and antagonists are the only data implicating external endogenous ATP in any physiological function in the cochlea.

Frank and Kossl (1996) hypothesized that a change in the set point of the cochlear amplifier will change the magnitude of the quadratic DPOAE in a direction opposite to that of the cubic DPOAEs. The shortening and lengthening of the outer hair cells (OHCs) is thought to be a part of the cochlear amplifier, while others suggest a role for the stereocilia in this process (Martin & Hudspeth, 1999; Ricci, 2001; Ricci, Wu, & Fettiplace, 1998). Deiters' cells appear to be positioned to directly affect the set point of the cochlear amplifier. Deiters' cells attach to the base of the OHCs, and their long stalks or phalangeal processes attach to the apex of OHCs (Slepecky, 1996). Therefore, OHCs work against the load applied by Deiters' cells. A change in the Deiters' cells' load would alter the set point of the cochlear amplifier. Deiters' cells have ATP receptors on their perilymph surface (Bobbin, Campbell, LeBlanc, & Lousteau, 2001; Dulon, 1995). This suggests that endogenous ATP released into perilymph may modulate cochlear mechanics by altering the mechanical properties of Deiters' cells (i.e., altering the load Deiters' cells apply to OHCs). If this hypothesis is correct, then the changes in cochlear mechanics (i.e., DPOAEs) evoked by chemicals such as ATP antagonists delivered into the perilymph may in part be due to the blockade of the actions of endogenous ATP on Deiters' cells (Bobbin et al., 1998, 2000). Deiters' cells are connected by gap junctions, so the actions of ATP probably involve a large number of Deiters' cells. In addition, there are ATP receptors on other cells in the cochlea such as Hensen's cells. Present evidence indicates those receptors are located on the endolymph surface of the cells (Bobbin et al., 1998, 2000; Lagostena, Ashmore, Kachar, & Mammano, 2001). However, in the future the hypotheses and model may have to be expanded to include additional cells such as Hensen's cells. The area certainly needs additional research.

Deiters' cells have curved stalks. The cytoskeleton (Slepecky, 1996) probably determines the degree of curvature. Dulon, Blanchet, and Laffon (1994) demonstrated that intracellular photoliberation of caged Ca^{2+} will decrease the curvature and increase the stiffness of the stalk or phalangeal process of isolated Deiters' cells. Therefore, experiments were carried out to test whether extracellular application of ATP to isolated Deiters' cells would induce a movement of their stalks. Results indicate that application of a depolarizing current, a hyperpolarizing current, and ATP induce a movement of the stalks of Deiters' cells providing additional evidence for the hypothesis. Portions of these results have been previously reported (Bobbin, 2001; Bobbin, LeBlanc et al., 2001).

MATERIALS AND METHODS

The care and use of the animals reported on in this study were approved by Louisiana State University Health Science Center's (LSUHSC's) Institutional Animal Care and Use Committee. Cells were isolated as previously described (Kujawa, Erostegui et al., 1994). Briefly, adult pigmented guinea pigs (300–500 g) were anesthetized with urethane (1.5 gm/kg, i.p.) and sacrificed by decapitation, and the bulla separated and placed in a modified Hank's balanced saline (HBS). The bone surrounding the cochlea was removed, and the organ of Corti was placed in 200 µl of HBS containing collagenase (1 mg/ml, Type IV, Sigma) for 1 to 10 min to increase cell dissociation. The cells were then mechanically isolated and transferred into the dishes containing HBS using a microsyringe. The HBS solutions contained (in mM): 137 or 127 NaCl, 5.36 KCl, 2.5 CaCl2, 0.5 MgCl2, 10 HEPES, 10 D-Glucose, 5 or 0 sucrose, 2 Na-pyruvate, 2 creatine, and 2 ascorbate. The pH was adjusted to 7.4 by the addition of appropriate amounts of NaOH. The osmolality of the two solutions was 287 (127 NaCl, 0 sucrose) and 308 (137 mM NaCl, 5 sucrose) mOsm/kg water as monitored by utilizing a freezing point osmometer (Precision Systems, model # 5002). The 285 mOsm HBS was used in some experiments on the assumption that healthy cells would autoregulate their volume, survive the dissection, and help in selecting only healthy cells for the experiments. Several morphological criteria were used to judge the viability and suitability of the cells used in the experiments. These included no visible movement of intracellular organelles, the appearance of normal turgor, an intact stalk, minimal cellular debris attached to the cell, and either the cell body or stalk attached to the bottom of the dish with the other end free to move. Occasionally, a Deiters' cell with an attached OHC was found and studied. The dishes were placed on an inverted microscope stage (Nikon Diaphot with Hoffman modulation contrast), and the cells were monitored with a video camera and simultaneously videotaped. All experiments were carried out at room temperature (25°C).

With the use of computer hardware (Data Translation DT 2853) and software (DT-IRIS), the tapes were analyzed for change in the position of the freely moving portion of the cell. A visually recognizable cellular landmark was followed along a set of X and Y coordinate values on the monitor. The measurements were taken from single frames selected from the final seconds of each 1-minute interval from the tape recordings. The largest or smallest coordinate value in the period of time over which the cell was measured was arbitrarily given a zero value. Since the movements of the tips of the stalks were not linear, a plot of the distance moved along each individual coordinate at 1-min intervals gave the best representation of the movement over time. The coordinate with the largest observed movement was used to calculate the mean ± s.e.m. The movements induced by high levels of anodal and cathodal current (50 to 1000 nA) were compared by calculating total accumulated movement for each without consideration of direction of movement. For this purpose, the distance between the landmark's momentary and original positions was measured and added to the previously measured distance moved. Calibration of the measurement system was performed using a calibrated reticulum. The smallest incremental distance resolved was 0.3 µm.

RESULTS AND DISCUSSION

Many cells studied had floppy stalks that moved in a jerky fashion in both directions about a given set point. Apparently, this movement was in response to the movement of the fluid in the dish. Other cells, floppy and not floppy, had stalks that slowly moved in one direction over a period of minutes (Figures 5–1 and 5–2). In other cells, the tip of the stalk seemed to oscillate from one position to another and back over a period of minutes. Cells were observed for varying periods of time to ensure that some degree of stability had been reached in the stalk movement before testing the effects of ATP or current. If no stability was attained, the cell was discarded.

The first set of experiments tested whether iontophoretic application of ATP from a delivery pipette would induce a movement of the stalks of Deiters' cells. The current was applied using an iontophoretic unit (WPI Model # 160) connected to a silver/chloride-coated silver wire inserted into the pipette and a second silver/chloride-coated silver wire placed in the bath. In this set of experiments, only low levels of current (10 to 50 nA) were used. An anodal current (pipette wire negative or the cathode) was used to iontophoretically eject ATP^{-2} ($ATPNa_2$;165 mM) from the pipette tip while the second wire in the bath was the anode. As a control, the anodal current was used to eject Cl^- (NaCl;165 mM). The tip of the pipette (1 to 5 µm in diameter) was placed approximately 2 to 5 µm from the cell body with the orifice directed at the place where it was thought the base of the OHC would have attached. The ejection current was applied in concurrent 1-min steps of 10, 20, 30, 40, and 50 nA. The stalk of Deiters' cells moved slowly in response to the iontophoretic application of ATP^{-2} (7 cells; Figure 5–3) and of Cl^- (7 cells). The cells were monitored for 5 to 10 min following the iontophoretic application, and some degree of recovery occurred during this time in a few cells. Surprisingly, no difference was noted between the responses induced by ATP^{-2} and Cl^- indicating that the current was the stimulus inducing the movement and not the ejected anion. Since the membrane in the region of the cathode will be depolarized by the current (as discussed on page 32 in Woodbury, 1965), it appears that a depolarization of the cell membrane induced the stalk to move. These results are surprising in that several authors have reported that Deiters' cells do not move in response to application of current (e.g., Brownell, Bader, Bertrand, & Ribaupierre, 1985; Dulon et al., 1994; Santos-Sacchi, 1989).

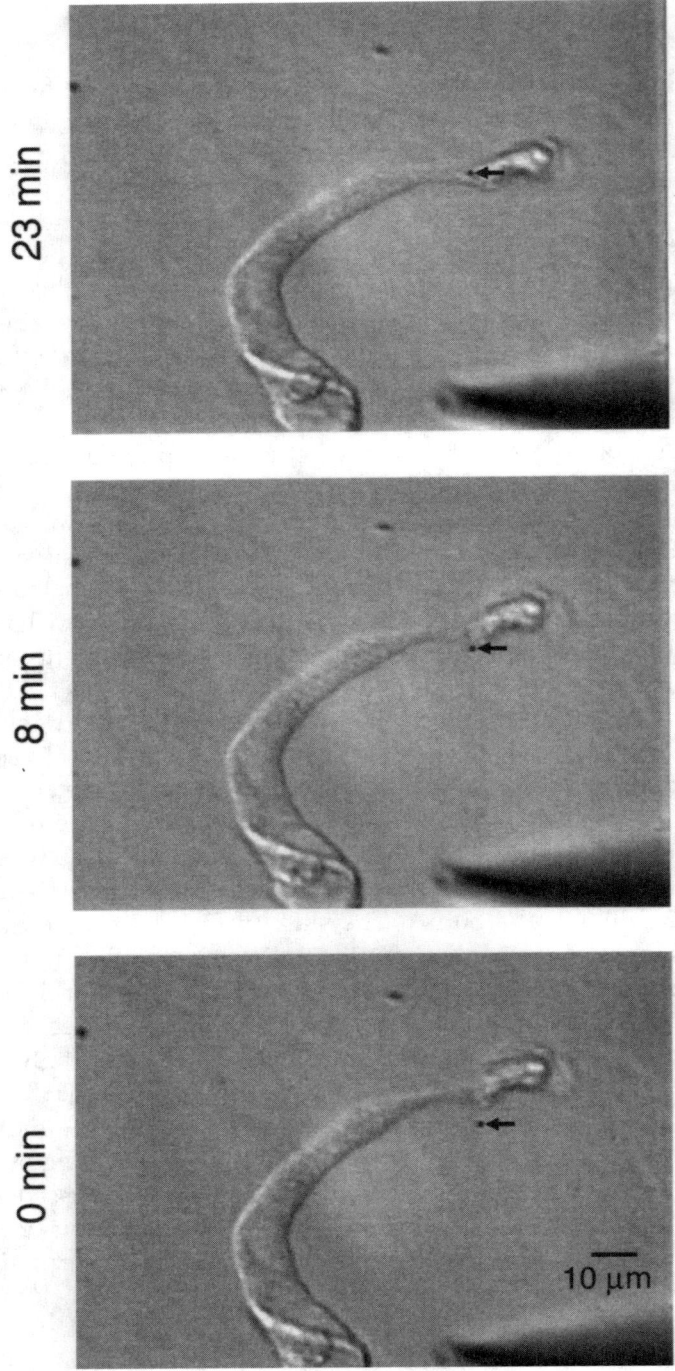

Figure 5–1. Example of a phalangeal process or stalk of a Deiters' cell slowly moving over time without an external stimulus being applied. Such cells were classified as unstable and were not tested. The black arrow is placed near the tip of the stalk to help visualize the movement over time. The time the frame was captured from the videotape is given over each frame.

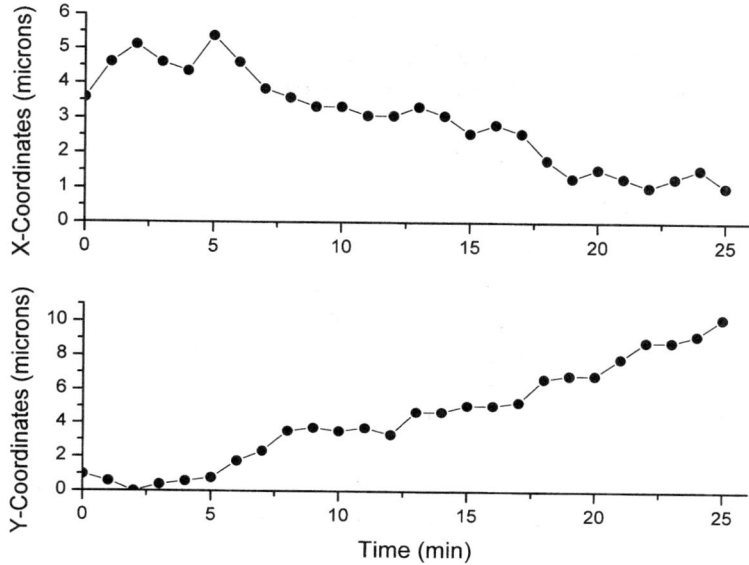

Figure 5–2. Measurement of the stalk movement shown in Figure 5–1 in terms of X and Y coordinates in microns.

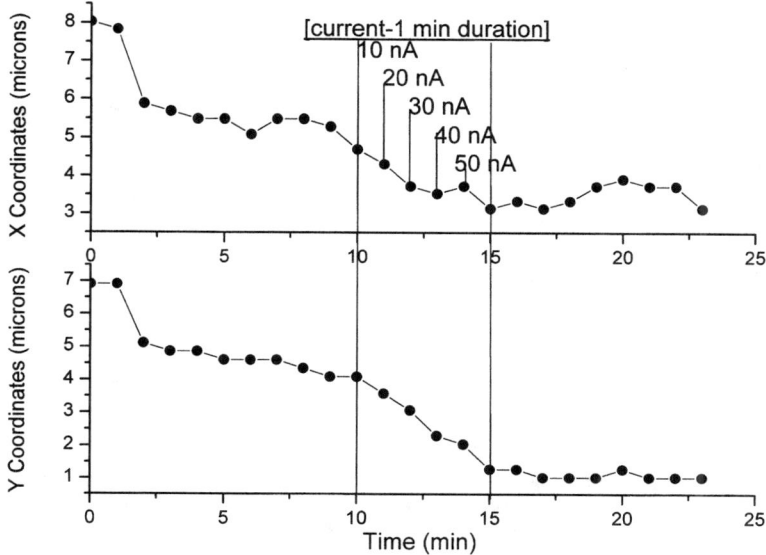

Figure 5–3. Low-level depolarization-induced movement of a Deiters' cell stalk. The extracellular anodal current (pipette wire negative or the cathode) was applied at increasing levels from 10 to 50 nA for durations of 1 min starting at 10 min.

Explanations for these negative results may be that in the present experiments the stimulus was applied for a longer period of time, and the movement of the cells was recorded over a longer time period than in previous studies.

Given these results with low levels of current, higher levels of current were tested to see if they would induce even greater stalk movement. In these high current (50 to 1,000 nA) experiments, the pipettes (NaCl; 0.5M) were tested both as the cathode (wire in the pipette negative or the cathode; anodal current; $n = 8$ cells) and as the anode (wire in the pipette positive or the anode; cathodal current; $n = 5$ cells). The current was applied in concurrent 2-min steps of 50, 100, 200, 400, and 1,000 nA. The tip of the pipette was placed very close to the cell near the nucleus. The stalk of the Deiters' cells moved slowly in response to the application of both types of currents. Extracellular anodal current (i.e., cell depolarization) induced movements of the stalks of Deiters' cells that altered the distance between the stalk and the cell body, with the final and largest movements those that increased the overall curvature of the cell (Figure 5–4). Cathodal current

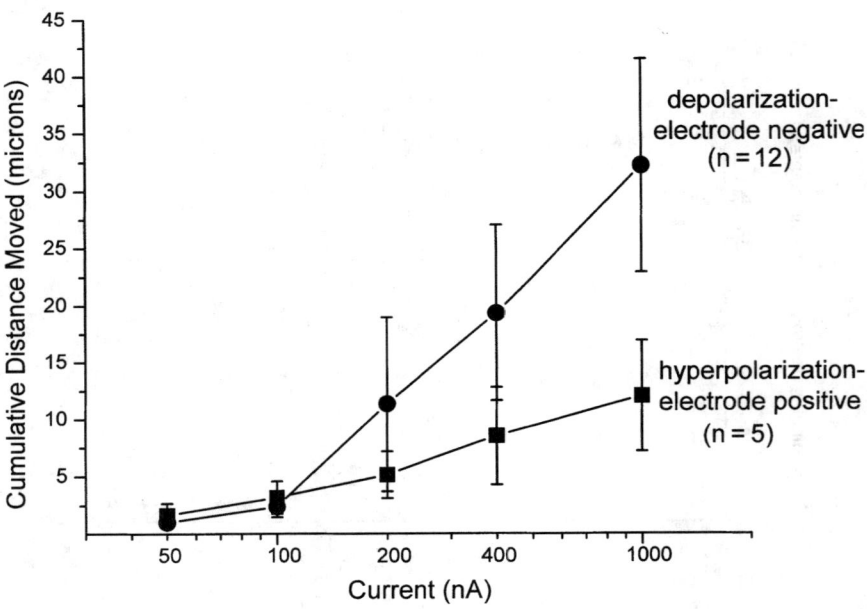

Figure 5–4. Cumulative movement of stalks of Deiters' cells (mean ± SE) induced by increasing steps of high levels of current (50, 100, 200, 400, and 1,000 nA). The currents were applied for 2 min at each level.

(cell hyperpolarization) was less effective than anodal current, and the movement induced was less than that induced by the anodal current (Figure 5–4). The average cumulative total distance moved as a function of current in several cells is shown in Figure 5–4. Figure 5–5 shows an example where the cell was first exposed to increasing levels of cathodal current application (50 to 1000 nA), and no movements were observed in the stalk (data not shown). Following this treatment, a large anodal current (−1000 nA) was applied. As shown, the stalk initially (10 sec) uncurled (moved away from the cell body) and then slowly curled toward the cell body. This treatment was followed by application of a large cathodal current (+1000 nA). Again, the stalk initially (before the 8 sec) curled (not shown) and then slowly uncurled. The volume of the cell increased as the stalk curled during the application of anodal current.

Others have reported movements of the organ of Corti to electrical stimulation (Richter, Rao, Koch, & Dallos, 2001) and to intense sound (Flock, Flock, Fridberger, Scarfone, & Ulfendahl, 1999; Fridberger, Flock, Ulfendahl, & Flock, 1998) that reduce the distance between the reticular lamina and the basilar membrane. The data presented here indicate that at least some of the movement observed in the whole organ of Corti may have been due to movements of the stalks of the Deiters' cells.

The movements observed in response to high level currents were accompanied by changes in size of the cell body. This may indicate that the electrical stimulus induced a transport of ions and water that changed the volume of the cell and caused the stalk to change its curvature. Arguing against this hypothesis is the fact that exposure of the cells to hypotonic solutions often caused a swelling that seemed to engulf the stalk rather than bend or curl the stalk as seen with electrical stimulation (data not shown). Alternatively, the bending of the fibers within the cell that control cell shape and stalk position may have pushed on the cell membrane. This could result in a widening of the cell body without a change in volume and give the appearance of an increase in cell volume. The mechanisms responsible for the stalk movement and the changes in the size of the cell body await further experimentation.

Since the application of ATP by iontophoresis failed to differentiate between ATP^- and the control (Cl^-), the drug application method was changed to pressure ejection from pipettes containing either 100 µM ATP dissolved in HBS or HBS alone. The solutions were applied for 10 sec and directed at the cell body where the base of the OHC was

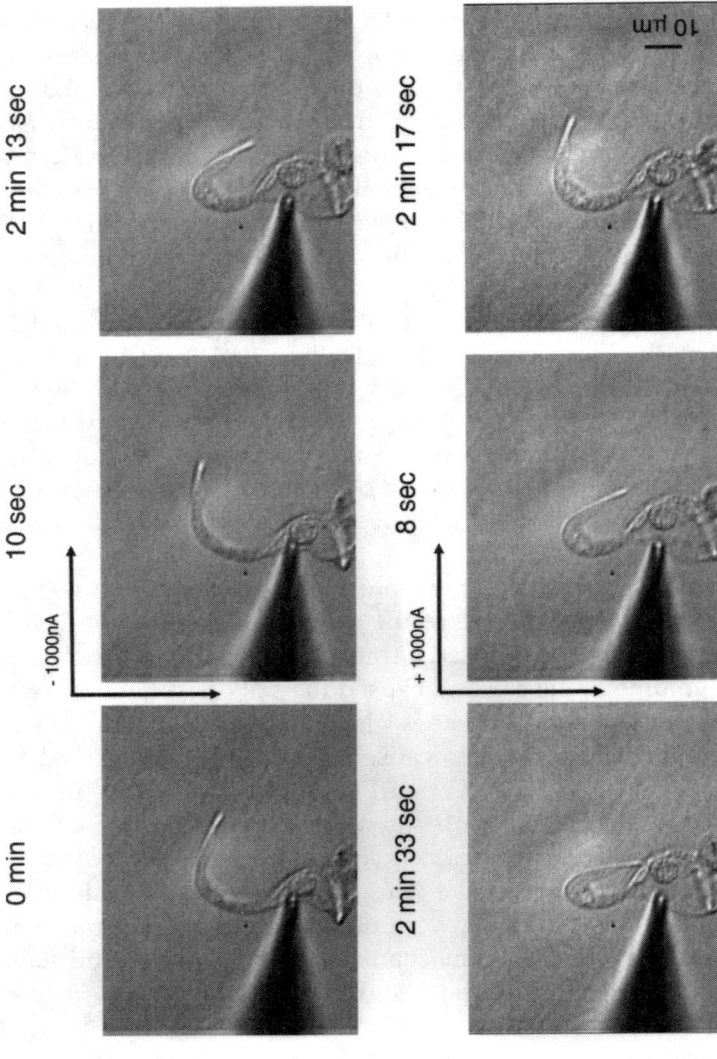

Figure 5–5. An example of a cell membrane depolarization (anodal current; pipette wire negative) induced movement of a stalk of a Deiters' cell and a hyperpolarization-induced (cathodal current; pipette wire positive) recovery. Shown are frames of the cell taken before (0 min) and various times after application of depolarization (10 sec, 2 min 13 sec, and 2 min 33 sec) and after application of hyperpolarization (8 sec, and 2 min 17 sec).

probably attached to the Deiters' cell. For these experiments, the bath containing the cell was perfused at 0.2 ml/min to wash away the applied drug. The HBS did not induce a movement of the stalks. On the other hand, the stalks of Deiters' cells moved slowly in response to the ATP (Figures 5–6 and 5–7). Future experiments will test lower concentrations of ATP and antagonists of ATP receptors.

The movements of the stalks of Deiters' cells induced by ATP support our hypothesis that the large changes in the cubic and quadratic distortion products induced by ATP agonists and antagonists in vivo are due, at least in part, to changes in the mechanical properties of

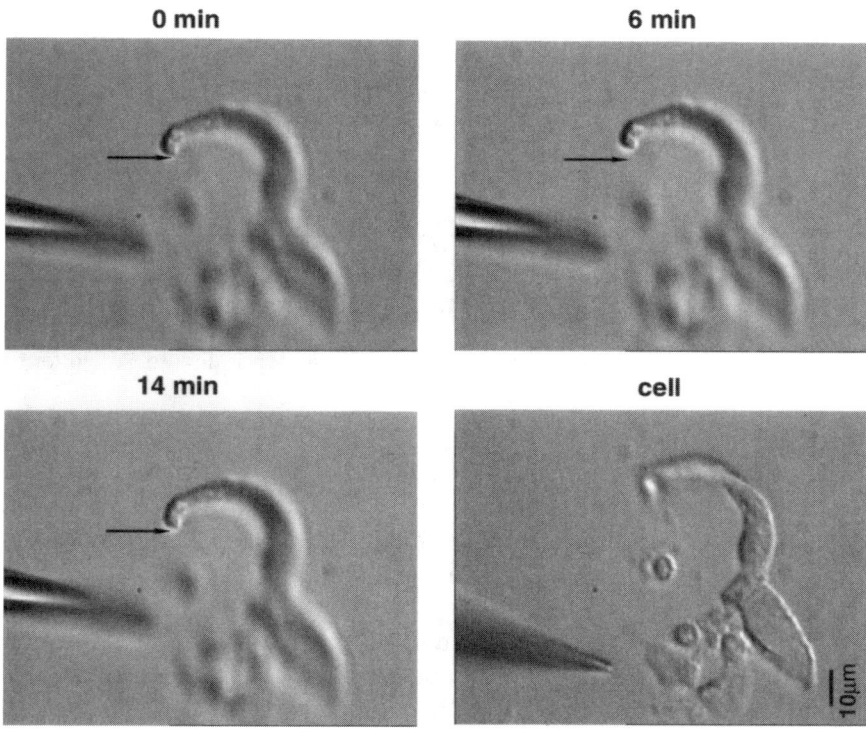

Figure 5–6. Example of a stalk of a Deiters' cell moving reversibly in response to 100 µM ATP applied by pressure puff for 10 sec from a pipette pointed at the cell body. Shown are frames of the cell taken before (0 min) application of the ATP, at the time after ATP application when maximal movement occurred (6 min), and at the time after application when recovery occurred (14 min). A frame focusing on the cell body (cell) is included to show the characteristic shape of Deiters' cells. The black arrow near the tip of the stalk is placed to help visualize the movement.

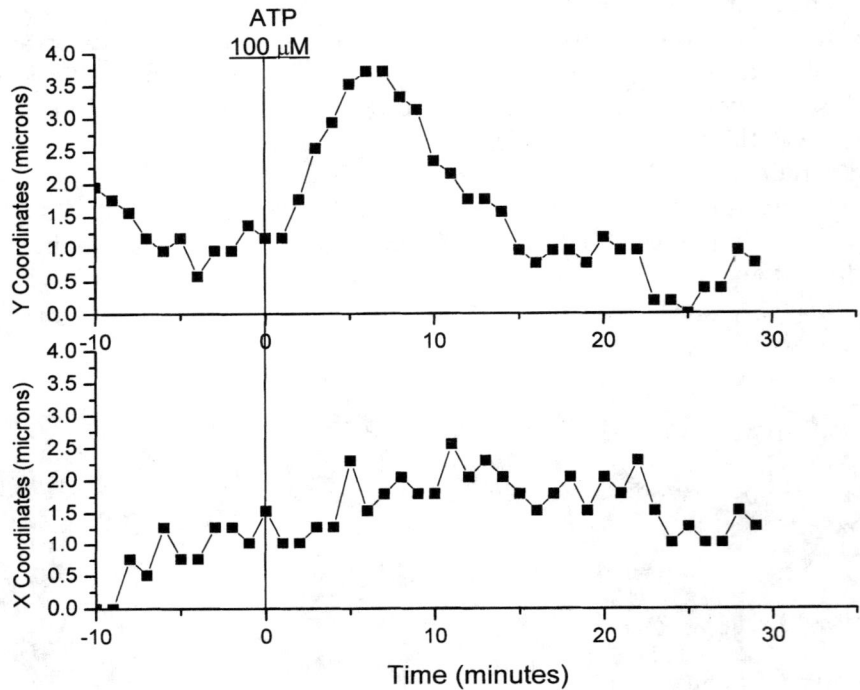

Figure 5–7. Measurement of the stalk movement shown in Figure 5–6 in terms of X and Y coordinates in microns.

Deiters' cells. These changes in Deiters' cells may then change the load on the OHCs and, in this manner, alter the set point of the operation of the cochlear amplifier (Bobbin et al., 1998, 2000; Chen et al., 1998; Kujawa, Erostegui et al., 1994; Kujawa, Fallon, & Bobbin, 1994; Skellett et al., 1997).

The molecular mechanisms underlying the Deiters' cell motion induced by ATP remain to be determined. Possible mechanisms include activation of ionotropic P2X receptors (Ashmore & Ohmori, 1990; Bobbin et al., 2000; Chen & Bobbin, 1998; Chen, LeBlanc, & Bobbin, 1997; Chen, Parker, Barnes, Deininger, & Bobbin, 2000; Chen et al., 1998; Dulon, 1995; Dulon, Moataz, & Mollard, 1993; Lagostena & Mammano, 2001; Skellett et al., 1997) and activation of metabotropic P2Y receptors (Matsunobu & Schacht, 2000; Moataz, Saito, & Dulon, 1992; Niedzielski & Schacht, 1992). Whether calcium plays any role in either the electrical or ATP induced movements of the stalks of Deiters' cells described in the present experiments remains to be determined.

SUMMARY AND MODEL

During the continuous presentation of primaries, the magnitude of sound-evoked quadratic DPOAE changes over time (e.g., Kujawa, Fallon, & Bobbin, 1995; Kujawa, Fallon, Skellett, & Bobbin, 1996). Both ATP antagonists, suramin and PPADS, alter the magnitude of the quadratic and the cubic DPOAEs and the change in magnitude of the quadratic DPOAE over time (Chen et al., 1998; Skellett et al., 1997). Agonists of ATP receptors also change DPOAEs magnitude (Kujawa, Erostegui et al., 1994). These observations form the experimental basis for the hypothesis that the magnitudes of these DPOAEs are influenced by endogenous, extracellular levels of ATP (Bobbin et al., 1998). We speculate further that this endogenous ATP is acting on Deiters' cells to alter the load on the OHCs, the proposed motors of the active process, changing their set point as modeled by Frank and Kossl (1996). The experiments described provide additional support for the hypothesis. In vivo, ATP may be released from unidentified adjacent cells (e.g., OHCs) or the nerve fibers forming synapses on Deiters' cells (Fechner, Burgess, Adams, Liberman, & Nadol, 1998) to induce a change in the mechanical properties of Deiters' cells as part of a feedback loop involving the adjacent cells and the Deiters' cells. The purpose of such a loop could be to provide a mechanism for the cochlea to maintain an optimal set point and gain of the cochlear amplifier in the presence of varying sound intensities. This adjustment may be reflected in the relative magnitudes of the cubic and quadratic DPOAEs.

Acknowledgments: Thanks to Anthony Ricci, PhD, for help and discussion. This work was supported in part by a research grant from National Science Foundation Grant IBN-9817165 and the American Hearing Research Foundation.

REFERENCES

Ashmore, J. F., & Ohmori, H. (1990). Control of intracellular calcium by ATP in isolated outer hair cells of the guinea-pig cochlea. *Journal of Physiology (London), 428,* 109–131.

Bobbin, R. P. (1996). Chemical receptors on outer hair cells and their molecular mechanisms. In C. I. Berlin (Ed.), *Hair cells and hearing aids* (pp. 29–55). San Diego, CA: Singular Publishing Group.

Bobbin, R. P. (1997). Transmitters in the cochlea: The chemical machinery in the ear. In C. I. Berlin (Ed.), *Neurotransmission and hearing loss: Basic science, diagnosis, and management* (pp. 25–46). San Diego, CA: Singular Publishing Group.

Bobbin, R. P. (2001). ATP induced motion of the stalks of isolated cochlear Deiters' cells. *NeuroReport, 12,* 1000–1004.

Bobbin, R. P., Barnes, P. A., Chen, C., Deininger, P., LeBlanc, C. S., & Parker, M. S. (2000). Transmitters in the cochlea: ATP as a neuromodulator in the organ of Corti. In C. I Berlin & B. Keats (Eds.), *Genetics and hearing loss* (pp. 87–110). San Diego, CA: Singular Publishing Group.

Bobbin, R. P., Campbell, J., LeBlanc, C. S., & Lousteau, S. (2001). Motion of the stalks of isolated Deiters' cells. *Association for Research in Otolaryngology Abstracts, 24,* 230.

Bobbin, R. P., Chen, C., Nenov, A. P., & Skellett, R. A. (1998). Transmitters in the cochlea: The quadratic distortion product and its time varying response may reflect the function of ATP in the cochlea. In C. I. Berlin (Ed.), *Otoacoustic emissions* (pp. 61–83). San Diego, CA: Singular Publishing Group.

Bobbin, R. P., LeBlanc, Mandhare, M., & Parker, M. S. (2001). Additional studies on the role of ATP as a neuromodulator in the organ of Corti. In C. I. Berlin & R. P. Bobbin (Eds.), *Hair cells: Micromechanics and hearing* (pp. 129–153). San Diego, CA: Singular Publishing Group.

Bobbin, R. P., & Thompson, M. H. (1978). Effects of putative transmitters on afferent cochlear transmission. *Annals of Otology, Rhinology, and Laryngology, 87,* 185–190.

Brownell, W. E., Bader, C .R., Bertrand, D., & de Ribaupierre, Y. (1985) Evoked mechanical responses of isolated cochlear outer hair cells. *Science, 227,* 194–196.

Chen, C., & Bobbin, R. P. (1998). P2X receptors in cochlear Deiters' cells. *British Journal of Pharmacology, 124,* 337–344.

Chen, C., LeBlanc, C., & Bobbin, R. P. (1997). Differences in the distribution of responses to ATP and acetylcholine between outer hair cells of rat and guinea pig. *Hearing Research, 110,* 87–94.

Chen, C., Parker, M. S., Barnes, P. A., Deininger, P., & Bobbin, R. P. (2000). Functional expression of three $P2X_2$ receptor splice variants from guinea pig cochlea. *Journal of Neurophysiology, 83,* 1502–1509.

Chen, C., Skellett, R. A., Fallon, M., & Bobbin, R. P. (1998) Additional pharmacological evidence that endogenous ATP modulates cochlear mechanics. *Hearing Research, 118,* 47–61.

Dulon, D. (1995). Ca^{2+} signaling in Deiters cells of the guinea-pig cochlea active process in supporting cells? In A. Flock, D. Ottoson, & M. Ulfendahl, (Eds.), *Active hearing* (pp. 195–207). Oxford, UK: Elsevier Science Ltd.

Dulon, D., Blanchet, C., & Laffon, E. (1994). Photo-released intracellular Ca^{2+} evokes reversible mechanical responses in supporting cells of the guinea-pig organ of Corti. *Biochemical and Biophysical Research Communications, 201,* 1263–1269.

Dulon, D., Moataz, R., & Mollard, P. (1993). Characterization of Ca^{2+} signals generated by extracellular nucleotides in supporting cells of the organ of Corti. *Cell Calcium, 14,* 245–254.

Fechner, F. P., Burgess, B. J., Adams, J. C., Liberman, M. C., & Nadol, J. B., Jr. (1998). Dense innervation of Deiters' and Hensens's cells persists after chronic deefferentation of guinea pig cochleas. *The Journal of Comparative Neurology, 400,* 299–309.

Flock, A., Flock, B., Fridberger, A., Scarfone, E., & Ulfendahl, M. (1999). Supporting cells contribute to control of hearing sensitivity. *Journal of Neuroscience, 19,* 4498–4507.

Frank, G., & Kossl, M. (1996). The acoustic two-tone distortions 2f1-f2 and f2-f1 and their possible relation to changes in the operating point of the cochlear amplifier. *Hearing Research, 98,* 104–115.

Fridberger, A., Flock, A., Ulfendahl, M., & Flock, B. (1998). Acoustic overstimulation increases outer hair cel Ca $^{2+}$ concentrations and causes dynamic contractions of the hearing organ. *Proceedings of the National Academy of Science, 95,* 7127–7132.

Housley, G. D. (1997). Extracellular nucleotide signaling in the inner ear. *Molecular Neurobiology, 16,* 21–48.

Housley, G. D., Kanjhan, R., Raybould, N. P., Greenwood, D., Salih, S. G., Jarlebark, L., Burton, L. D., Setz, V. C. M., Cannell, M. B., Soeller, C., Christie, D. L., Usami, S., Matsubara, A., Yoshie, H., Ryan, A. F., & Thorne, P. R. (1999). Expression of the $P2X_2$ receptor subunit of the ATP-gated ion channel in the cochlea: Implications for sound transduction and auditory neurotransmission. *Journal of Neuroscience, 19,* 8377–8388.

Kujawa, S. G., Erostegui, C., Fallon, M., Crist, J., & Bobbin, R. P. (1994). Effects of adenosine 5'-triphosphate and related agonists on cochlear function. *Hearing Research, 76,* 87–100.

Kujawa, S. G., Fallon, M., & Bobbin, R. P. (1994). ATP antagonists cibacron blue, basilen blue and suramin alter sound-evoked responses of the cochlea and auditory nerve. *Hearing Research, 78,* 181–188.

Kujawa, S. G., Fallon, M., & Bobbin, R. P. (1995). Time-varying alterations in the f_2-f_1 DPOAE response to continuous primary stimulation. I. Response characterization and contribution of the olivocochlear efferents. *Hearing Research, 85,* 142–154.

Kujawa, S. G., Fallon, M., Skellett, R. A., & Bobbin, R. P. (1996). Time-varying alterations in the f_2-f_1 DPOAE response to continuous primary stimulation. II. Influence of local calcium-dependent mechanisms. *Hearing Research, 97,* 153–164.

Lagostena, L., Ashmore, J. F., Kachar, B., & Mammano, F. (2001). Purinergic control of intercellular communication between Hensen's cells of the guinea-pig cochlea. *Journal of Physiology (London), 531.3,* 693–706.

Lagostena, L., & Mammano, F. (2001). Intracellular calcium dynamics and membrane conductance changes evoked by Deiters' cell purinoceptor activation in the organ of Corti. *Cell Calcium, 29,* 191–196.

Martin, P., & Hudspeth, A. J. (1999) Active hair-bundle movements can amplify a hair cell's response to oscillatory mechanical stimuli. *Proceedings of the National Academy of Sciences, USA, 96,* 14306–14311.

Matsunobu, T., & Schacht, J. (2000). Nitric oxide/cyclic GMP pathway attenuates ATP-evoked intracellular calcium increase in supporting cells of the guinea pig cochlea. *Journal of Comparative Neurology, 423,* 452–461.

Moataz, R., Saito, T., & Dulon, D. (1992). Evidence for voltage sensitive Ca^{2+} channels in supporting cells of the organ of Corti: Characterization by indo-1 fluorescence. *Advances in the Biosciences, 83,* 53–59.

Munoz, D. J. B., Kendrick, I.S., Rassam, M., & Thorne, P. R. (2001). Vesicular storage of adenosine triphosphate in the guinea-pig cochlear lateral wall and concentrations of ATP in the endolymph during sound exposure and hypoxia. *Acta Otolaryngology, 121,* 10–15.

Niedzielski, A. S., & Schacht, J. (1992). P2 purinoceptors stimulate inositol phosphate release in the organ of Corti. *NeuroReport 3,* 273–275.

Parker, M. S., Larroque, M., Campbell, J. M., Bobbin, R.P., & Deininger, P. (1998). Novel variant of the P2X2 ATP receptor from guinea pig organ of Corti. *Hearing Research, 121,* 62–70.

Ricci, A. J. (2001). Fast transducer adaptation, physiological implications and underlying mechanisms. In C. I. Berlin and R. P. Bobbin (Eds.), *Hair cells: Micromechanics and hearing* (pp. 45–66). San Diego, CA: Singular Publishing Group.

Ricci, A. J., Wu, Y. C., & Fettiplace, R. (1998). The endogenous calcium buffer and the time course of transducer adaptation in auditory hair cells. *Journal of Neuroscience, 18,* 8261–8277.

Richter, C. P., Rao, R., Koch, D. B., & Dallos, P. (2001). Electrical stimulation in the hemicochlea: Cell integrity and current distribution. *Association for Research in Otolaryngology Abstracts, 24,* 230.

Santos-Sacchi, J. (1989). Asymmetry in voltage-dependent movements of isolated outer hair cells from the organ of Corti. *Journal of Neuroscience, 9,* 2954–2962.

Skellett, R. A., Chen, C., Fallon, M., Nenov, A. P., & Bobbin, R. P. (1997). Pharmacological evidence that endogenous ATP modulates cochlear mechanics. *Hearing Research, 111,* 42–54.

Slepecky, N. B. (1996). Structure of the mammalian cochlea. In P. Dallos, A . N. Popper, & R. R. Fay (Eds.), *The Cochlea* (pp. 44–129). New York: Springer-Verlag.

Woodbury, J. W. (1965). Action potential: Properties of excitable membranes. In T. C. Ruch, H. D. Patton, J. W. Woodbury, & A. L. Towe (Eds.), *Neurophysiology* (pp. 26–72). Philadelphia: W.B. Saunders.

Xiang, Z., Bo, X., & Burnstock, G. (1999). P2X receptor immunoreactivity in the rat cochlea, vestibular ganglion and cochlear nucleus. *Hearing Research, 128,* 190–196.

Usher Syndrome Genes

Sevtap Savas, PhD
Bronya J. B. Keats, PhD
Department of Genetics
Louisiana State University Health Sciences Center
New Orleans, Louisiana

INTRODUCTION

The Usher syndromes (USH) are a group of both genetically and clinically heterogeneous disorders (reviewed in Keats & Corey, 1999). The main tissues affected are the retina, the vestibular organ, and the hair cells of the organ of Corti in the inner ear. Degeneration of the hair cells underlies the hearing loss observed in USH. Vestibular dysfunction results in balance problems and delayed motor development in some patients with USH. Retinitis pigmentosa (RP) in USH results from the degeneration of the rod photoreceptors in the retina. The RP starts as night blindness and may progress to total blindness. Other clinical findings in patients with USH include olfactory loss, structural anomalies of nasal cilia, and decreased sperm motility (Arden & Fox, 1979; Hunter, Fishman, Mehta, & Kretzer, 1986; Marietta et al., 1997; Zrada, Braat, Doty, & Laties, 1996).

Three clinical types of USH (USH1-3) have been defined based on age of onset, severity of the symptoms, and presence of vestibular dysfunction. USH1 is the most severe form of the disease. It is characterized by severe to profound hearing loss across all frequencies. Hearing aids are not helpful for patients with USH1, but cochlear implants for these patients are often successful (Hinderlink, Brokx, Mens, & van den Broek, 1994; Young, Hohnson, Mets, & Hain, 1995). Complete loss of vestibular function distinguishes USH1 from the other clinical forms of the disease. In addition, RP tends to be more severe in patients with USH1, with onset during childhood.

USH2 is a less severe form of the disease in which the hearing loss is moderate to severe. Vestibular function is normal in patients with USH2, and RP starts in the third or fourth decade of life. USH3 is distinguished from the other two types by the progressive nature of the hearing loss. The degree of vestibular dysfunction, as well as the age of onset of retinal degeneration, is variable in USH3.

All types of USH are inherited in an autosomal recessive pattern. The frequency of USH is estimated to be 2 to 6 per 100,000 in different populations (Boughman, Vernon, & Shaver, 1983; Hope, Bundey, Prrops, & Fielder, 1997; Rosenberg, Haim, Hauch, & Parving, 1997; Tamayo et al., 1991). On average, USH accounts for 4% of congenital deafness, 18% of pigmentary retinopathy, and more than 50% of deaf-blindness. The prevalence of USH2 is reported to be higher than USH1 (Kimberling et al., 1995; Rosenberg et al., 1997), with USH3 being the rarest form of the disease.

GENETICS OF USHER SYNDROMES

Six different USH1 genes have been localized to chromosomal regions and four (USH1B, USH1C, USH1D, USH1F) have been identified. The genes responsible for USH1A and USH1E have not yet been isolated. USH1A was mapped to chromosome 14q in families from the Poitou-Charentes region of Western France (Kaplan et al., 1992); the interval was refined (Larget-Piet et al., 1994) and analyzed for candidate genes (Eudy et al., 1997). A single family with USH1E (a consanguineous Moroccan family) has been mapped to chromosome 21q11.2-22.1 (Chaib et al., 1997). USH1D and USH1F are both on chromosome 10, and Astuto et al. (2000) suggested that there may be a third gene in the USH1D/USH1F region.

To date, three USH2 genes have been localized to specific chromosomal regions, but so far only the USH2A gene has been characterized. USH2B has been mapped in a Tunisian family to chromosome 3p23-24.2, a region that overlaps with a nonsyndromic deafness locus, DFNB6 (Honani et al., 1999). It is not known if USH2B and DFNB6 are allelic or due to abnormalities in two different genes in this region. USH2C is characterized by less severe RP (onset almost a decade later than USH2A and USH2B) and has been mapped to chromosome 5q (Pieke-Dahl et al., 2000).

The only USH3 locus reported so far is on chromosome 3q21-q25 (Sankila et al., 1995). It was mapped in Finnish families, and the frequency of USH3 in this population is relatively high (Joensuu et al., 1996). A few families with USH3 from Sweden (Kimberling et al., 1995), Italy (Gasparini, De Fazio, Croce, Stanziale, & Zelante, 1998) and Spain (Espinos et al., 1998) have also been reported; all show linkage to the 3q21-q25 chromosomal region. Recently, a bacterial artificial chromosome (BAC) contig spanning the USH3 critical region was constructed, and two candidate genes mapping to this bacterial artificial chromosome (BAC) were excluded as the USH3 gene (Joensuu, Hamalainen, Lehesjoki, de la Chapelle, & Sankila, 2000).

Three atypical families with RP, severe sensorineural hearing loss, and enamel hypoplasia have been defined (Innis, Sieving, McMillan, & Weatherly, 1998; Pieke-Dahl et al., 2000), and linkage to any of the USH loci could be excluded in two of these families (Pieke-Dahl et al., 2000). Thus, at least one, and probably more, USH loci are yet to be localized and identified.

USH1B

Approximately 75% of patients with USH1 have USH1B (Astuto et al., 2000; Weil et al., 1995). Families with USH1B from several different countries were found to be linked to markers on chromosome 11q15.3 (Kimberling et al., 1992; Smith et al., 1992). Bonne-Tamir et al. (1994) refined the critical USH1B region by analyzing a large Samaritan kindred. Later, the gene (MYO7A) encoding an unconventional myosin VIIa protein was identified as the USH1B gene (Weil et al., 1995). This gene consists of 48 exons and is expressed in a variety of tissues including retina and cochlea. Myosin VIIa moves on cytoplasmic actin filaments (Weil et al., 1995) and contains domains similar to those that cause membrane association, suggesting that it may be involved in membrane trafficking (Hasson, 1997). Mutations in the orthologous mouse gene (myo7a) cause the deafness mutant *shaker-1* (Gibson et al., 1995). Moreover, forms of autosomal recessive (DFNB2) and autosomal dominant (DFNA12) nonsyndromic deafness are also due to mutations in the MYO7A gene (Liu, Walsh, Mburu et al., 1997; Liu, Walsh, Tamagawa et al., 1997).

USH1C

USH1C was first described in the Acadian population of Louisiana (Kloepfer, Laguaite, & McLaurin, 1966), and the USH1C gene was mapped to chromosome 11p15.1 in Acadian families (Smith et al., 1992). Later, families with USH1 from Pakistan and Lebanon were also reported to be linked to the same region, indicating that USH1C is not restricted to the Acadian population (Bitner-Glindzicz et al., 2000; Saouda et al., 1998; Verpy et al., 2000). After delineation of the interval containing the USH1C gene, subsequent analyses were conducted to refine it and to construct physical maps across the USH1C critical region (Ayyagari, Smith, Pelias, & Hejtmancik, 1995; DeAngelis et al., 1998; Keats, Nouri, Pelias, Deininger, & Litt, 1994). Recently, the USH1C gene was shown to encode a PDZ-domain containing protein called harmonin (Bitner-Glindzicz et al., 2000; Verpy et al., 2000). Several PDZ-domain proteins in a variety of organisms have been characterized, and these domains are thought to be involved in cell-signaling processes (reviewed in Fanning & Anderson, 1999).

So far, six different mutations in USH1C have been reported (Bitner-Glindzicz et al., 2000; Verpy et al., 2000; Zwaenepoel et al., 2001). All of these mutations reside in the 5' end of the gene and result in either abnormalities in splicing or premature termination of translation. In Acadian patients with USH1C, a 216G>A substitution in exon 3 leads to the creation of a cryptic splice site. As a result, 13 amino acids from the first PDZ-domain of harmonin are deleted, and the resulting transcript is unstable (Bitner-Glindzicz et al., 2000). Our preliminary computational analyses suggest that this internally deleted PDZ-domain is still recognized as a PDZ-domain. The most frequent mutation in the USH1C gene is a 238-239insC mutation in exon 3, which has been detected in Pakistanis, Europeans, and, surprisingly, in a single Acadian patient with USH1C (Bitner-Glindzicz et al., 2000; Verpy et al., 2000; Zwaenepoel et al., 2001). Haplotype analysis suggests that this mutation may have a single common ancestor (Zwaenepoel et al., 2001). Finally, Bitner-Glindzicz et al. (2000) also described siblings with a partial deletion of USH1C in a contiguous deletion syndrome characterized by hyperinsulinism, enteropathy, deafness, and retinitis pigmentosa. Interestingly, while the absence of harmonin is associated with enteropathy, this condition is not observed in patients with USH1C.

Verpy et al. (2000) reported the presence of a variable number of tandem repeat (VNTR) polymorphism residing in intron 5 of the USH1C gene. This 45 bp VNTR was found in 2, 3, 4, 6, and 8 repeat sizes in a control population consisting of French individuals. Acadian patients with USH1C, however, were found homozygous for 9 repeats. In addition, a sequence difference was detected in these patients. The last repeat of all observed alleles in the control sample contained a "t" nucleotide at the eighth position in the VNTR sequence, while the previous repeats had a "g" at the same position. In contrast, the Acadian USH1C allele had the "t" nucleotide at that position in the last two repeats. We have analyzed this VNTR in six different populations and a total of 400 unrelated individuals. Our results show that the Acadian USH1C VNTR allele is restricted to the Acadian USH1C population. We have also shown that this 9-repeat VNTR allele and the 216G>A mutation in exon 3 are in complete disequilibrium in this population, which is consistent with previous haplotype analysis (Keats et al., 1994). It is not known whether this particular VNTR allele is linked to the pathogenesis of this disease in the Acadian population, as suggested by Verpy et al. (2000).

USH1D

USH1D was first mapped in a Pakistani family to chromosome 10q (Wayne et al., 1996). Two groups recently identified the USH1D gene (Bolz et al., 2001; Bork et al., 2001). They showed that it is composed of 69 exons and is expressed in retina, cochlea, brain, kidney, skeletal muscle, blood, and pancreas. Preliminary studies suggest alternative splicing of this gene, although the physiological relevance of this finding is not known (Bork et al., 2001). The amino acid sequence of the protein encoded by the USH1D gene predicts 27 extracellular cadherin repeats; thus the gene is named CDH23. Cadherins are a large protein family, which contain extracellular calcium binding domains and are involved in intercellular adhesion. Analyses of families with USH1D from Pakistan (Bork et al., 2001), Cuba, and Germany (Bolz et al., 2001) resulted in the detection of nonsense, splice site, and missense mutations, as well as a 3 bp deletion, in affected individuals. Interestingly, in the Cuban family, although all the affected individuals had congenital deafness, the RP was variable, ranging from a mild to a severe course. Genotype-phenotype correlation studies in this family showed that the mildly affected individuals were homozygous for a missense mutation, while the severely affected were homozygous for a splice site mutation. The compound heterozygotes manifested variable severity of the RP. Bork et al. (2001) also identified six different missense mutations in the CDH23 gene in two Indian and three Pakistani families with DFNB12, a locus for nonsyndromic recessive deafness that had previously been mapped to the same region as USH1D (Chaib et al., 1996).

USH1F

USH1F was mapped in an inbred Hutterite family to chromosome 10 (Wayne et al., 1997). A protocadherin gene, Pcdh15, which is responsible for a hearing loss (Ames waltzer) phenotype in mouse was recently characterized, and the human ortholog was mapped to chromosome 10 (Alagramam et al., 2001). Subsequent analyses revealed the presence of splice site and nonsense mutations in the PCDH15 gene in two families from Pakistan with USH1F (Ahmed et al., 2001). PCDH15 has 11 extracellular calcium binding domains, and it is the second cadherin-like gene mutated in Usher syndromes. Protocadherins belong to the cadherin protein superfamily and are possibly involved in the process that enables neurons to recognize their synaptic partners (Shapiro & Colman, 1999).

USH2A

USH2A accounts for about 70% of all USH cases (Kimberling et al., 1995). In families with mostly European ancestors, linkage analysis localized the USH2A gene on chromosome 1q41 (Kimberling et al., 1995). Later, isolated families with USH2A from Norway (a Saami family) and the Cayman Islands were also linked to this locus (Fagerheim et al., 1999). Subsequent studies, including the construction of a yeast artificial chromosome (YAC) contig across the USH2A region (Sumegi et al., 1996), and refinement of the critical region (Bessant, Payne, Plant, Bird, & Bhattacharya, 1998), helped to isolate the disease gene, which is expressed in adult and fetal retina as well as fetal cochlea (Eudy et al., 1998). The gene encodes a novel protein (usherin) that contains both laminin epidermal growth factor and fibronectin type II motifs and shows homology with extracellular matrix and cell-cell adhesion proteins.

There are several identified mutations in the USH2A gene (Dreyer et al., 2000; Eudy et al., 1998; Liu et al., 1999; Weston et al., 2000). The most frequent mutation is a one base pair deletion (2299delG, formerly known as 2314delG) leading to a shift in the reading frame and premature termination of translation. Analysis of intragenic polymorphisms suggests that all patients with the 2299delG mutation are probably descended from a single common ancestor (Dreyer et al., 2000; Dreyer et al., 2001).

Liu et al. (1999) described monozygotic twins who were both homozygous for the 2299delG mutation but showed variation in severity of symptoms. The same study revealed the homozygous 2299delG mutation in members of three families from the United

Kingdom and China with an atypical USH2A phenotype characterized by progressive hearing loss, vestibular dysfunction, and RP.
Thus, other genetic and/or environmental factors must be contributing to the phenotype in at least some cases of USH.

Rivolta, Sweklo, Berson, and Dryja (2000) examined patients
diagnosed with autosomal recessive RP and found a novel missense
(Cys759Phe) mutation in the USH2A gene in 4.5% of cases. A compound heterozygote for this mutation and 2299delG did not have
hearing loss. In contrast, several of these patients were heterozygous
for the 2299delG but did not have the Cys759Phe mutation, and most
of them reported mild hearing loss. These findings demonstrate that
mutations in USH2A may cause recessive RP with minimal hearing
loss as well as Usher syndrome type 2A.

USH2 has been diagnosed in a few Acadian families. In one of
these families, Eudy et al. (1998) found that the patients were heterozygous for a two base pair deletion (4338-9delCT). So far the mutation on the other chromosome has not been detected. Thus, we do not
yet know if the USH2A gene is responsible for Acadian USH2.

SUMMARY

The Usher syndromes are a group of devastating disorders characterized by dual sensory loss. Understanding the molecular basis of this
disease is important in order to (a) ease the symptoms and the psy-
chological burden experienced by the families, (b) make carrier testing
possible, (c) confirm the clinical diagnosis, and (d) develop gene-
based therapies. So far, a total of 10 genes involved in the development
of USH have been mapped to chromosomal regions, and 5 of them
have been characterized (USH1B, USH1C, USH1D, USH1F, USH2A).
Functional studies of the USH genes identified are consistent with the
disorder being a result of abnormalities in the cytoskeletal/signal
transduction components in the affected tissues.

Observations that some atypical patients with USH carry the
same mutations as typical patients with USH, and that the same mutation may result in different phenotypes, suggest the involvement of
other genetic and/or environmental factors in the development
of USH. Considering the characterized/presumed functions of the
USH proteins described so far, speculation that these USH proteins
physically or functionally interact with each other is valid. In fact,
Adato et al. (1999) analyzed a family with both USH3 and USH1 phe-

notypes and suggested a possible interaction between MYO7A and the protein encoded by the USH3 gene. Involvement of non-USH modifier genes in these phenotypic variations is also likely.

REFERENCES

Adato, A., Kalinski, H., Weil, D., Chaib, H., Korostishevsky, M., & Bonne-Tamir, B. (1999). Possible interaction between USH1B and USH3 gene products as implied by apparent digenic deafness inheritance. *American Journal of Human Genetics, 65,* 261–265.

Ahmed, Z. M., Riazuddin, S., Bernstein, S. L., Ahmed, Z., Khan, S., Griffith, A. J., Morell, R. J., Friedman, T. B., Riazuddin, S., & Wilcox, E. R. (2001). Mutations of the protocadherin gene PCDH15 cause Usher syndrome type 1F. *American Journal of Human Genetics, 69,* 25–34.

Alagramam, K. N., Murcia, C. L., Kwon, H. Y., Pawlowski, K. S., Wright, C. G., & Voychik, R. P. (2001). The mouse Ames waltzer hearing-loss mutant is caused by mutation of Pcdh15, a novel protocadherin gene. *Nature Genetics, 27,* 99–102.

Arden, G. B., & Fox, B. (1979). Increased incidence of abnormal nasal cilia in patients with retinitis pigmentosa. *Nature, 279,* 534–536.

Astuto, L. M., Weston, M. D., Carney, C. A., Hoover, D. M., Cremers, C. W. R. J., Wagenaar, M., Moller, C., Smith, R. J. H., Pieke-Dahl, S., Greenberg, J., Ramesar, R., Jacobson, S. G., Ayuso, C., Heckenlively, J. R., Tamaya, M., Gorin, M. B., Reardon, W., & Kimberling, W. J. (2000). Genetic heterogeneity of Usher syndrome: Analysis of 151 families with Usher type I. *American Journal of Human Genetics, 67,* 1569–1574.

Ayyagari, R., Li, Y., Smith, R. J., Pelias, M. Z., & Hejtmancik, J. F. (1995). Fine mapping of the Usher syndrome type IC to chromosome 11p14 and identification of flanking markers by haplotype analysis. *Molecular Vision, 1,* 2.

Bessant, D. A., Payne, A. M., Plant, C., Bird, A. C., & Bhattacharya, S. S. (1998). Further refinement of the Usher 2A locus at 1q41. *Journal of Medical Genetics, 35,* 773–774.

Bitner-Glindzicz, M., Lindley, K. J., Rutland, P., Blaydon, D., Smith, V. V., Milla, P. J., Hussain, K., Furth-Lavi, J., Cosgrove, K. E., Shepherd, R. M., Barnes, P. D., O'Brien, R. E., Farndon, P. A., Sowden, J., Liu, X-Z., Scanlan, M. J., Malcolm, S., Dunne, M. J., Aynsley-Green, A., & Glaser, B. (2000). A recessive contiguous gene deletion syndrome causing infantile hyperinsulinism, enteropathy and deafness identifies the Usher type 1C gene. *Nature Genetics, 26,* 56–60.

Bolz, H., von Brederlow, B., Ramirez, A., Bryda, E. C., Kutsche, K., Nothwang, H. G., Seeliger, M., del C.-Salcedo Cabrera, M., Vila, M. C., Molina, O. P., Gal, A., & Kubisch, C. (2001). Mutation of CDH23, encoding a new member of the cadherin gene family, causes Usher syndrome type 1D. *Nature Genetics, 27,* 108–112.

Bonne-Tamir, B., Korostishevsky, M., Kalinsky, H., Seroussi, E., Beker, R., Weiss, S., & Godel, V. (1994). Genetic mapping of the gene for Usher syndrome: Linkage analysis in a large Samaritan kindred. *Genomics, 20,* 36–42.

Bork, J. M., Peters, L. M., Riazuddin, S., Bernstein, S. L., Ahmed, Z. M., Ness, S. L., Polomeno, R., Ramesh, A., Schloss, M., Srikumari Srisailpathy, C. R., Wayne, S., Bellman, S., Desmukh, D., Ahmed, Z., Khan, S. N., Der Kaloustian, V. M., Li, X. C., Lalwani, A., Riazuddin, S., Bitner-Glindzicz, M., Nance, W. E., Liu, X-Z., Wistow, G., Smith, R. J. H., Griffith. A. J., Wilcox, E. R., Friedman, T. B., & Morell, R. J. (2001). Usher syndrome 1D and nonsyndromic autosomal recessive deafness DFNB12 are caused by allelic mutations of the novel cadherin-like gene CDH23. *American Journal of Human Genetics, 68,* 26–37.

Boughman, J. A., Vernon, M., & Shaver, K. A. (1983). Usher syndrome: Definition and estimate of prevalence from two-high risk populations. *Journal of Chronic Diseases, 36,* 595–603.

Chaib, H., Place, C, Salem, N., Dode, C. M., Chardenoux, S., Weissenbach, J., El Zir, E., Loiselet, J., & Petit, C. (1996). Mapping of DFNB12, a gene for a non-syndromal autosomal recessive deafness, to chromosome 10q21-22. *Human Molecular Genetics, 5,* 1061–1064.

Chaib, H., Kaplan, J., Gerber, S., Vincent, C., Ayadi, H., Slim, R., Munnich, A., Weissenbach, J., & Petit, C. (1997). A newly identified locus for Usher syndrome type I, USH1E, maps to chromosome 21q21. *Human Molecular Genetics, 6,* 27–31.

DeAngelis, M. M., Doucet, J. P., Drury, S., Sherry, S. T., Robichaux, M. B., Den, Z., Pelias, M. Z., Ditta, G. M., Keats, B. J., Deininger, P. L., & Batzer, M. A. (1998). Assembly of a high-resolution map of the Acadian Usher syndrome region and localization of the nuclear EF-hand acidic gene. *Biochimica et Biophysica Acta, 1407,* 84–91.

Dreyer, B., Tronebjaerg, L., Rosenberg, T., Weston, M. D., Kimberling, W. J., & Nilssen, O. (2000). Identification of novel USH2A mutations: Implication for the structure of USH2A protein. *European Journal of Human Genetics, 8,* 500–506.

Dreyer, B., Tranebjaerg, L., Brox, V., Rosenberg, T., Moller, C., Beneyto, M., Weston, M. D., Kimberling, W. J., & Nilssen, O. (2001). A common ancestral origin of the frequent and widespread 2299delG USH2A mutation. *American Journal of Human Genetics, 69,* 228–234.

Espinos, C., Najera, C., Millan, J. M., Ayuso, C., Baiget, M., Perez-Garrigues, H., Rodrigo, O., Vilela, C., & Beneyto, M. (1998). Linkage analysis in Usher syndrome type I (USH1) families from Spain. *Journal of Medical Genetics, 35,* 391–398.

Eudy, J. D., Ma-Edmonds, M., Yao, S. F., Talmadge, C. B., Kelley, P. M., Weston, M. D., Kimberling, W. J., & Sumegi, J. (1997). Isolation of a novel human homologue of the gene encoding for echinoderm microtubule-associated protein (EMAP) from the Usher syndrome type 1a locus at 14q32. *Genomics, 43,* 104–106.

Eudy, J. D., Weston, M. D., Yao, S., Hoover, D. M., Rehm, H. L., Ma-Edmonds, M., Yan, D., Ahmad, I., Cheng, J. J., Ayuso, C., Cremers, C., Davenport, S., Moller, C., Talmadge, C. B., Beisel, K. W., Tanaya, M., Morton, C. C., Swaroop, A., & Kimberling, W. J. (1998). Mutation of a gene encoding a protein with extracellular matrix motifs in Usher syndrome type IIa. *Science, 280,* 1753–1757.

Fagerheim, T., Raeymaekers, P., Merren, J., Mani, K., Jha, G. K., Baumbach, L., Brox, V., Breines, E., Holdo, B. E., & Tranebjaerg, L. (1999). Homozygosity mapping to USH2a locus in two isolated populations. *Journal of Medical Genetics, 36,* 144–147.

Fanning, A. S., & Anderson, J. M. (1999). Protein modules as organizers of membrane structure. *Current Opinion in Cell Biology, 11,* 432–439.

Gasparini, P., De Fazio, A., Croce, A. I., Stanziale, P., & Zelante, L. (1998). Usher syndrome type III (USH3) linked to chromosome 3q in an Italian family. *Journal of Medical Genetics, 35,* 666–667.

Gibson, F., Walsh, J., Mburu, P., Varela, A., Brown, K. A., Antonio, M., Beisel, K. W., Steel, K. P., & Brown, S. D. M. (1995). A type VII myosin encoded by the mouse deafness gene Shaker-1. *Nature, 374,* 62–64.

Hasson, T. (1997). Unconventional myosins, the basis for deafness in mouse and man. *American Journal of Human Genetics, 61,* 801–805.

Hinderlink, J. B., Brokx, J. P., Mens, L. H., & van den Broek, P. (1994). Results from four cochlear implant patients with Usher's syndrome. *Annals of Otology, Rhinology, and Laryngology, 103,* 285–293.

Honani, M., Ghorbel, A., Boulila-Elgaied, A., Ben Zina, Z., Kammaun, W., Drira, M., Chaabouni, M., Petit, C., & Ayadi, H. (1999). A novel locus for Usher syndrome type II, USH2B, maps to chromosome 3 at p23-24.2. *European Journal of Human Genetics, 7,* 363–367.

Hope, C. I., Bundey, S., Prrops, D., & Fielder, A. R. (1997). Usher syndrome in the city of Birmingham—prevalence, and clinical classification. *The British Journal of Ophthalmology, 81,* 46–53.

Hunter, D. G., Fishman, G. A., Mehta, R. S., & Kretzer, F. L. (1986). Abnormal sperm and photoreceptor axonemes in Usher's syndrome. *Archives d'ophtalmologie, 104,* 385–389.

Innis, J. W., Sieving, P. A., McMillan, P., & Weatherly, P. A. (1998). Apparently new syndrome of sensorineural hearing loss, retinal pigment epithelium lesions and discolored teeth. *American Journal of Medical Genetics, 75,* 13–17.

Joensuu, T., Blanco, G., Pakarinen, L., Sistonen, P., Kaariainen, H., Brown, S., de la Chapelle, A., & Sankile, E. M. (1996). Refined mapping of the Usher syndrome type III locus on chromosome 3, exclusion of candidate genes, and identification of the putative mouse homologous region. *Genomics, 38,* 255–263.

Joensuu, T., Hamalainen, R., Lehesjoki, A-E., de la Chapelle, A., & Sankila, E-M. (2000). A sequence-ready map of the Usher syndrome type III critical region on chromosome 3q. *Genomics, 63,* 409–416.

Kaplan, J., Gerber, S., Bonneau, D., Rozet, J., Delrieu, O., Briard, M., Dollfus, H., Ghazi, I., Dufier, J., Frezal, J., & Munnich, A. (1992). A gene for Usher syndrome type I (USH1) maps to chromosome 14q. *Genomics, 14*, 979–988.

Keats, B. J. B., Nouri, N., Pelias, M. Z., Deininger, P. L., & Litt, M. (1994). Tightly linked flanking microsatellite markers for the Usher syndrome type I locus on the short arm of chromosome 11. *American Journal of Human Genetics, 54*, 681–686.

Keats, B. J. B., & Corey, D. P. (1999). The Usher syndromes. *American Journal of Medical Genetics, 89*, 158–166.

Kimberling, W. J., Moller, C. G., Davenport, S., Priluck, I. A., Beighton, P. H., Greenberg, J., Reardon, W., Weston, M. D., Kenyon, J. B., Grunkmeyer, J. A., Pieke Dahl, S., Overbeck, L. D., Blackwood, D. J., Brower, A. M., Hoover, D. M., Rowland, P., & Smith, R. J. H. (1992). Linkage of Usher syndrome type I gene (USH1B) to the long arm of chromosome 11. *Genomics, 14*, 988–994.

Kimberling, W. J., Weston, M. D., Moller, C., van Aarem, A., Cremers, C. W. R. J., Sumegi, J., Ing, P. S., Connolly, C., Martini, A., Milani, M., Tamayo, M. L., Bernal, J., Greenberg, J., & Ayuso, C. (1995). Gene mapping of Usher syndrome type IIa. Localization of the gene to a 2.1-cM segment of chromosome 1q41. *American Journal of Human Genetics, 56*, 216–223.

Kloepfer, H. W., Laguaite, J. K., & McLaurin, J. W. (1966). The hereditary syndrome of congenital deafness and retinitis pigmentosa (Usher's syndrome). *Laryngoscope, 76*, 850–862.

Larget-Piet, D., Gerber, S., Bonneau, D., Rozet, J. M., Marc, S., Ghazi, I., Dufier, J. L., David, A., Bitoun, P., Weissenbach, J., Munnich, A., & Kaplan, J. (1994). Genetic heterogeneity of Usher type 1 in French families. *Genomics, 21*, 138–143.

Liu, X-Z., Hope, C., Liang, C. Y., Zou, J. M., Xu, L. R., Cole, T., Mueller, R. F., Bundey, S., Nance, W., Steel, K. P., & Brown, S. D. M. (1999). A mutation (2314delG) in the Usher syndrome type IIa gene: High prevalence and phenotypic variation. *American Journal of Human Genetics, 64*, 1221–1225.

Liu, X. Z., Walsh, J., Mburu, P., Kendrick-Jones, J., Cope, M. J. T. V., Steel K. P., & Brown S. D. M. (1997). Mutations in the myosin VIIA gene cause non-syndromic recessive deafness. *Nature Genetics, 16*, 188–190.

Liu, X. Z., Walsh, J., Tamagawa, Y., Kitamura, K., Nishizawa, M., Steel, K. P., & Brown, S. D. M. (1997). Autosomal dominant non-syndromic deafness (DFNA11) caused by a mutation in the myosin VIIA gene. *Nature Genetics, 17*, 268–269.

Marietta, J., Walters, K. S., Burgess, R., Ni, L., Fukushima, K., Moore, K. C., Hejtmancik, J. F., & Smith R. J. (1997). Usher's syndrome type IC: Clinical studies and fine-mapping of the disease locus. *The Annals of Otology, Rhinology, and Laryngology, 106*, 123–128.

Pieke-Dahl, S., Moller, C. G., Kelley, P. M., Astuto, L. M., Cremers, C. W. R. J., Gorin, M. B., & Kimberling, W. J. (2000). Genetic heterogeneity of Usher syndrome type II: Localization to chromosome 5q. *Journal of Medical Genetics, 37*, 256–262.

Rivolta, C., Sweklo, E. A., Berson, E. L., & Dryja, T. P. (2000). Missense mutation in the USH2A gene: Association with recessive retinitis pigmentosa without hearing loss. *American Journal of Human Genetics, 66,* 1975–1978.

Rosenberg, T., Haim, M., Hauch, A. M., & Parving, A. (1997). The prevalence of Usher syndrome and other retinal dystrophy-hearing impairment associations. *Clinical Genetics, 51,* 314–321.

Sankila, E. M., Pakarinen, L., Kaariainen, H., Aittomaki, K., Karjalainen, S., Sistonen, P., & de la Chapelle, A. (1995) Assignment of an Usher syndrome type III (USH3) gene to chromosome 3q. *Human Molecular Genetics, 4,* 93–98.

Saouda, M., Mansour, A., Bou Moglabey, Y., El Zir, E., Mustapha, M., Chaib, H., Nehme, A., Megarbane, A., Loiselet, J., Petit, C., & Slim, R. (1998). The Usher syndrome in the Lebanese population and further refinement of the USH2A candidate region. *Human Genetics, 103,* 193–198.

Shapiro, L., & Colman, D. R. (1999). The diversity of cadherins and implications for a synaptic adhesive code in the CNS. *Neuron, 23,* 427–430.

Smith, R. J. H., Lee, E. C., Kimberling, W. J., Daiger, S. P., Pelias, M. Z., Keats, B. J. B., Jay, M., Bird, A., Reardon, W., Guest, M., Ayyagari, R., & Hejtmancik, J. F. (1992). Localization of two genes for Usher syndrome type 1 to chromosome 11. *Genomics, 14,* 995–1002.

Sumegi, J., Wang, J. Y., Zhen, D. K., Eudy, J. D., Talmadge, C. B., Li, B. F., Berglund, P., Weston, M. D., Yao, S. F., Ma-Edmonds, M., Overbeck, L., Kelley, P. M., Zaborovsky, E., Uzvolgyi, E., Stanbridge, E. J., Klein, G., & Kimberling, W.J. (1996). The construction of a yeast artificial chromosome (YAC) contig in the vicinity of the Usher syndrome type IIa (USH2A) gene in 1q41. *Genomics, 35,* 79–86.

Tamayo, M. L., Bernal, J. E., Tamayo, G. E., Frias, J. L., Alvira, G., Vergara, O., Rodriguez, V., Uribe, J. I., & Silva, J. C. (1991). Usher syndrome: Results of a screening program in Colombia. *Clinical Genetics, 40,* 304–311.

Verpy, E., Leibovici, M., Zwaenepoel, I., Liu, X-Z., Gal, A., Salem, N., Mansour, A., Blanchard, S., Kobayashi, I., Keats, B. J. B., Slim, R., & Petit, C. (2000). A defect in harmonin, a PDZ domain-containing protein expressed in the inner ear sensory hair cells, underlies Usher syndrome type 1C. *Nature Genetics, 26,* 51–55.

Wayne, S., Der Kalaoustian, V. M., Schloss, M., Polomeno, R., Scott, D. A., Hejtmancik, J. F., Sheffiled, V. C., & Smith, R. J. (1996). Localization of the Usher syndrome type Id gene (USH1D) to chromosome 10. *Human Molecular Genetics, 5,* 1689–1692.

Wayne, S., Lowry, R. B., McLeod, D. R., Knaus, R., Farr, C., & Smith, R. J. H. (1997). Localization of the Usher syndrome type IF (USH1F) to chromosome 10. *American Journal of Human Genetics, 61*(Suppl.), A300.

Weil, D., Blanchard, S., Kaplan, J., Guilford, P., Gibson, F., Walsh, J., Mburu, P., Varela, A., Levilliers, J., Weston, M. D., Kelley, P. M., Kimberling, W. J., Wagenaar, M., Levi-Acobas, F., Larget-Piet, D., Munnich, A., Steel, K. P., Brown, S. D. M., & Petit, C. (1995). Defective myosin VIIA gene responsible for the Usher syndrome type 1B. *Nature, 374,* 60–61.

Weston, M. D., Eudy, J. D., Fujita, S., Yao, S. F., Usami, S., Cremers, C., Greenburg, J., Ramesar, R., Martini, A., Moller, C., Smith, R. J., Sumegi, J., & Kimberling, W. J. (2000). Genomic structure and identification of novel mutations in Usherin, the gene responsible for Usher syndrome type IIa. *American Journal of Human Genetics, 66,* 1199–1210.

Young, N. M., Hohnson, J. C., Mets, M. B., & Hain, T. C. (1995). Cochlear implants in young children with Usher's syndrome. *Annals of Otology, Rhinology, and Laryngology, 166,* 342–345.

Zrada, S. E., Braat, K., Doty, R. L., & Laties, A. M. (1996). Olfactory loss in Usher syndrome: Another sensory deficit? *American Journal of Medical Genetics, 64,* 602–603.

Zwaenepoel, I., Verpy, E., Blanchard, S., Meins, M., Apfelstedt-Sylla, E., Gal, A., & Petit, C. (2001). Identification of three novel mutations in the USH1C gene and detection of thirty-one polymorphisms used for haplotype analysis. *Human Mutation, 17,* 34–41.

Clinical Applications of Otoacoustic Emissions

Linda J. Hood, PhD
Charles I. Berlin, PhD
Kresge Hearing Research Laboratory
Department of Otorhinolaryngology
Louisiana State University Health Sciences Center
New Orleans, Louisiana

INTRODUCTION

The reports of transient evoked otoacoustic emissions (OAEs) by Kemp (1978); the motile characteristics of outer hair cells (OHCs) (Brownell, Bader, Bertrand, & de Ribaupierre, 1985); and the non-linear, sharply tuned vibration patterns of the basilar membrane (Khanna & Leonard, 1982) were each revolutionary discoveries in hearing science. Scientists gained important insight into cochlear processes, and clinicians acquired a sensitive new tool for use in distinguishing among various types of hearing disorders.

Otoacoustic emissions are widely used in humans and animals to study cochlear function and the efferent system. The origin of otoacoustic emissions is ascribed to processes associated with the mechanical motion of the OHCs, and OAEs are thought to be modulated by the efferent auditory pathways via the olivocochlear system (Kemp, 1978; Kemp & Chum, 1980). OAEs appear sensitive to subtle changes in cochlear function that are not revealed in the octave interval behavioral audiogram (e.g., Glattke & Kujawa, 1991; Martin, Probst, & Lonsbury-Martin, 1990; Ohlms, Lonsbury-Martin, & Martin,

1990; Probst, Lonsbury-Martin, & Martin, 1991). Otoacoustic emissions have high test-retest reliability, which contributes to their clinical utility (Berlin et al., 1991; Engdahl, Arnensen, & Mair, 1994; Roede, Harris, Probst, & Xu, 1993).

There are several types of OAEs that fit into two broad categories: spontaneous emissions and evoked otoacoustic emissions. Spontaneous OAEs are recorded in the absence of external stimuli and, as with other OAEs, are associated with normal cochlear function. Evoked OAEs are categorized as transient, distortion product, and stimulus frequency otoacoustic emissions. Transient evoked and distortion product OAEs are the most widely used clinically.

Transient OAEs are elicited by brief pulses (clicks) or tonebursts while distortion product OAEs are recorded in response to pairs of tones. The presence of transient and distortion product OAEs is consistent with cochlear sensitivity that is usually but not always either normal or in the mild hearing loss range. OAEs are affected by middle ear dysfunction related to attenuation of the stimulus signal and, probably more important, conduction of the low-level otoacoustic emission outward from the cochlea through the middle ear system.

OTOACOUSTIC EMISSIONS IN CLINICAL POPULATIONS

OAEs provide physiological information about cochlear function, and normal OAEs are believed to be related to OHC integrity. Thus, OAEs are useful in differentiating OHC from other disorders and are a valuable cross-check to other components of the audiological test battery. Based on the objectivity of the measure, OAEs also are useful in the evaluation of patients with suspected functional hearing loss.

Otoacoustic Emissions and Cochlear Hearing Loss

OAEs provide information about the presence or absence of greater than a mild cochlear hearing loss affecting the OHCs and are usually but not always associated with pure-tone thresholds better than 30 to 35 dB HL. OAEs also can provide insight into the configuration of a hearing loss based on presence or absence of OAEs in specific frequency regions. While OAEs can differentiate normal hearing and mild hearing losses from more severe hearing losses, they have not been found to accurately predict behavioral pure tone thresholds.

OAEs provide a valuable procedure for newborn hearing screening based on the objectivity of the measure and relative ease of administration. As a screening measure, OAEs are used to differentiate significant cochlear hearing loss from normal or nearly normal OHC function. It must be remembered, however, that OAEs are a physiological test of hair cell integrity and not a direct test of hearing. OAEs are often normal in the presence of neural hearing loss or inner hair cell (IHC) loss, as discussed in the next section.

Otoacoustic Emissions and Neural Hearing Loss

Otoacoustic emissions may or may not be present in patients with space-occupying lesions affecting the VIIIth nerve and/or caudal brainstem. Some patients with such neural lesions demonstrate an absence of OAEs, most likely due to restriction of blood flow to the cochlea, which limits the oxygen and nutrients needed by the cochlea (Robinette & Durrant, 1997). In addition to the effects on blood supply, neural lesions may destroy cochlear fibers by pressure, atrophy, or invasion and contribute to biochemical degradation of the fluids of the inner ear (Prasher, Tun, Brookes, & Luxon, 1995), thus affecting hair cell and other cochlear processes.

Patients with auditory neuropathy (perhaps more descriptively named auditory dys-synchrony) present with normal OAEs, barring any middle ear problems or other peripheral hearing loss. Normal OAEs occur in conjunction with neural dys-synchrony as documented by the absence of a synchronous auditory brainstem response (ABR), and the absence of middle ear muscle reflexes (MEMR) despite normal tympanometry (Berlin, Hood, Cecola, Jackson, & Szabo, 1993; Starr, Picton, Sininger, Hood, & Berlin, 1996). The presence of cochlear microphonics also is consistent with normal OHC function, and these responses are best measured by comparing averages obtained using positive versus negative polarity clicks (Berlin et al., 1998). Patients with auditory neuropathy/dys-synchrony generally show no masking level difference, which is consistent with abnormalities in processing of timing and phase information. Speech recognition is quite variable though generally much poorer than expected and is generally poor in noise or with competing messages. Patients also may lack a full complement of IHCs (Amatuzzi et al., 2001).

OTOACOUSTIC EMISSIONS AND EFFERENT FUNCTION

Central control is exercised on the auditory periphery via two efferent auditory reflexes. The MEMR controls the stapedius and tensor tympani muscles of the middle ear and the olivocochlear reflex (OCR) controls portions of the cochlea. Liberman and Guinan (1998) provide a valuable review of the properties of these reflexes and their roles in modifying auditory function.

Efferent Reflexes

The MEMR is characterized by binaural contraction of the stapedius muscles to loud sound and just prior to vocalization. The MEMR is mediated by the reflex arc from the cochlear branch of the VIIIth nerve via the brainstem to the facial VIIth nerve that innervates the stapedius muscle. The stapedius muscle reflex is measured clinically to assess middle ear function and the integrity of the neural reflex arc.

Cochlear function is modified via efferent pathways involving the fibers of the olivocochlear bundle as a component of the OCR. Auditory efferent fibers travel from the olivocochlear bundle at the level of the olivary complex in the brainstem through the vestibulocochlear (VIIIth) nerve to the cochlea. The medial olivocochlear fibers terminate primarily on the OHCs while the lateral olivocochlear fibers terminate mainly on primary auditory neurons at the base of the IHCs (Warr & Guinan, 1978; Warr, Guinan, & White, 1986). The OCR can be measured using test paradigms in which OAEs are altered through the introduction of a suppressor stimulus. Changes to emissions in the presence of a suppressor stimulus are thought to be modulated through the efferent auditory pathways via the olivocochlear system (Kemp, 1978; Kemp & Chum, 1980). Some possible functions of the OCR may be related to improved auditory sensitivity, improved listening in noise, and/or a protective function.

EFFERENT SUPPRESSION OF OTOACOUSTIC EMISSIONS

Several studies described suppression of spontaneous and transient evoked otoacoustic emissions in humans with normal auditory function (Berlin, Hood, Wen et al., 1993; Berlin, Hood, Hurley, Wen, & Kemp, 1995; Collet et al., 1990; Grose, 1983; Hood, Berlin, Hurley,

Cecola, & Bell, 1996; Mott, Norton, Neely, & Warr, 1989; Rabinowitz & Widen, 1984; Ryan, Kemp, & Hinchcliffe, 1991; Schloth & Zwicker, 1983; Veuillet, Collet, & Duclaux, 1991). The effects of contralateral stimuli on distortion product OAEs appear more variable, with reports of both increases and decreases in distortion product OAE amplitude with presentation of contralateral stimuli (Chery-Croze, Collet, & Morgon, 1993; Moulin, Collet, & Duclaux, 1993; Moulin, Collet, & Morgon, 1993; Nieschall, Beneking, & Stoll, 1997; Timpe-Syverson & Decker, 1999).

Efferent suppression of transient-evoked OAEs can be recorded by introducing a suppressor stimulus into the same, opposite, or both ears. In the contralateral suppression mode, a continuous noise is presented to the opposite ear during the time that the emission is recorded and averaged. This is the most commonly used method to study efferent suppression and perhaps the easiest and most rapid way to study the effect. However, binaural suppressor stimuli result in larger suppression effects than contralaterally presented suppressors (Berlin et al., 1995). A forward masking paradigm is employed when presenting a suppressor stimulus to the same ear from which the transient OAE is recorded to avoid unwanted interactions between the OAE-evoking stimulus and the suppressor stimulus. Procedural considerations in recording and analyzing suppression of OAEs are discussed in several sources (Berlin et al., 1995; Hood et al., 1996; Hood, Berlin, Goforth-Barter, Bordelon, & Wen, 1999).

Characteristics of Suppression of Transient OAEs in Normal Individuals

Suppression is characterized as a reduction in amplitude and/or time changes or phase shifts of emission peaks (e.g., Berlin, Hood, Cecola, et al., 1993; Berlin, Hood, Hurley, & Wen, 1994; Berlin, Hood, Wen et al., 1993; Collet et al., 1990; Ryan et al., 1991). Suppression amplitude varies among subjects though, in our experience, all normal subjects show efferent suppression in some time periods. Some of the characteristics of suppression are briefly summarized here. The characteristics of suppression in normal subjects are reviewed in detail in many of the cited articles and chapters.

Suppression is greatest in the 8 to 18 msec time period and in the lower frequencies (e.g., Berlin, Hood, Cecola et al., 1993; Berlin et al., 1994; Berlin, Hood, Wen et al., 1993; Collet et al., 1990; Hood et al.,

1996; Veuillet et al., 1991). Some normal subjects, who appear to have little or no suppression when a single value is calculated to represent the entire 20.48 msec period, show quantifiable suppression in the 8 to 18 msec range or in shorter specified time periods.

Suppression is proportionately greater for lower intensity stimuli than for higher intensity stimuli (Hood et al., 1996; Ryan & Kemp, 1996; Veuillet et al., 1991). Hood et al. (1996) observed greater suppression for click stimuli presented at 55–60 dB peak SPL than for 65 dB peak SPL clicks. Greater suppression for lower rather than higher intensity stimuli is consistent with function of the cochlear active process. This observation also reduces concern about the influence of acoustic cross-talk or middle ear muscle reflex interference since these factors should not exert greater effects at lower intensities.

Suppression of transient OAEs is greater for binaural suppressors than for ipsilateral or contralateral noise, and contralateral noise is the least effective suppressor (Berlin et al., 1995). This finding suggests that the preponderance of literature using only contralateral suppressors underestimates the overall efferent effect.

Age Effects on Suppression of Transient OAEs

Efferent suppression is present in some but not all infants with a higher incidence of suppression in term than preterm infants (Goforth et al., 2000; Hildesheimer, Hamburger, Ari-Even Roth, Muchnik, & Kuint, 1999; Morlet, Collet, Salle, & Morgon, 1993; Ryan & Piron, 1994). In addition, the Morlet et al. (1999) comparison of contralateral transient OAE suppression in right and left ears in 24 neonates indicated higher suppression values in the right than left ears of infants older than 36 weeks gestational age. This effect was not present in younger neonates, suggesting the gradual onset of functional asymmetries in the infant auditory system that may contribute to functional auditory lateralization in adults.

Transient OAE suppression decreases in older adults (Castor, Veuillet, Morgan, & Collet, 1994; Hood, Hurley, Goforth, Bordelon, & Berlin, 1997). Hood et al. (1997) compared the effects of binaural, ipsilateral, and contralateral suppressors on transient OAE suppression in subjects from 10 to 81 years. A gradual decline in suppression was observed across the age span and, of particular interest, greater reductions occurred for binaural than for ipsilateral or contralateral suppressor stimuli.

Relation of Suppression to Listening in Noise

Several investigators have suggested that one role of the efferent system may relate to the ability to distinguish signals in the presence of noise. While studies are just beginning in this area, there is some preliminary evidence to support this suggestion. Two such studies, by Micheyl, Carbonnel, and Collet (1995) and Micheyl, Morlet, Giraud, Collet, and Morton (1995), associate transient OAE suppression amplitude with thresholds for detection in noise and loudness adaptation, respectively.

Efferent Suppression in Cochlear Hearing Loss

Efferent suppression of OAEs is difficult to study in patients with greater than mild cochlear hearing losses because emissions are usually not present when hearing thresholds exceed 30–40 dB HL. Liang, Liu, and Liu (1997) measured contralateral suppression of transient OAEs with broadband noise in 24 ears with cochlear hearing loss. They reported that transient OAE amplitude and suppression of emissions were significantly reduced in patients with cochlear hearing loss in comparison to normal ears.

Efferent Suppression in Neural Disorders

Potential clinical value of measures of efferent function is demonstrated by observations that patients with certain types of neural disorders do not demonstrate normal efferent responses.

Patients with auditory neuropathy/dys-synchrony differ from those with radiologically or surgically documented space-occupying or other lesions of the VIIIth nerve. Auditory neuropathy/dys-synchrony patients show normal computed tomography (CT) and magnetic resonance imaging (MRI) results. Disruption of suppression of OAEs is observed in both patients with auditory neuropathy/dys-synchrony and patients with space-occupying lesions.

The presence of space-occupying lesions at the level of the VIIIth nerve and/or caudal brainstem can affect otoacoustic emissions and efferent suppression. In those patients where OAEs are present, it is possible to study efferent suppression. An interesting finding, reported in several studies, has been a consistent lack of or reduction in efferent suppression in these patients, suggesting that the efferent pathway is vulnerable to the effects of the lesion (Liang et al., 1997; Maurer, Beck, Mann, & Mintest, 1992; Prasher, Ryan, & Luxon, 1994).

Patients with auditory neuropathy consistently demonstrate the presence of OAEs but consistently show no or minimal suppression of transient OAEs for binaural, ipsilateral, and contralateral suppressor stimuli (Berlin, Hood, Cecola et al., 1993; Hood et al., 2000; Starr et al., 1991, 1996). In patients with bilateral auditory neuropathy, the lack of suppression of OAEs makes it difficult to separate possible contributions of afferent and efferent pathways. Patients with unilateral neuropathy can shed light on this question. Our observations in a unilateral auditory neuropathy patient indicate that the efferent system is functioning even for the neuropathy ear and can be partially activated by noise to the normal ear. However, when the neuropathy ear is stimulated, no efferent function in either ear is recordable.

Patients who undergo vestibular neurectomy provide an opportunity to confirm the effects of efferent suppression. Retrolabyrinthine neurectomy involves sectioning of the inferior vestibular fibers that carry both medial and lateral efferent bundles, with the goal of alleviating vertigo while preserving the afferent auditory fibers and cochlear function. Vestibular neurectomy patients demonstrated a reduction or lack of OAE suppression with contralateral noise in the operated ear while suppression was present in the unoperated ear (Giraud, Collet, Chery-Croze, Magnan, & Chays, 1995; Williams, Brooks, & Prasher, 1993, 1994). The large reduction in suppression observed in the operated ears of the vestibular neurectomy patients is consistent with the requirement for intact olivocochlear efferent fibers to obtain a full suppressive effect.

Efferent Suppression in Other Clinical Patients

Berlin, Hood, Goforth-Barter, and Bordelon (1999) reported increased efferent suppression in some patients with hyperacusis who complained that ordinary sounds were loud and frequently intolerable. In some ears of these patients and in some patients who did not demonstrate inordinately large efferent suppression bilaterally, a digression from the normal pattern of greater suppression for binaural than ipsilateral or contralateral suppression was also observed. In addition, some of these patients showed asymmetric suppression patterns between the two ears despite symmetry in behavioral responses. Berlin et al. (1999) suggest that this may represent an apparent failure of the efferent system to adapt input signals that may provide insight into some of the mechanisms underlying abnormal sensitivity to sound.

Several authors have suggested a possible role of the efferent system in the generation of tinnitus. Suppression of both transient and distortion product OAEs is reduced in ears with tinnitus compared to nontinnitus ears in patients with unilateral tinnitus as well as in patients with bilateral tinnitus compared to control subjects (Ceranic, Prasher, Raglan, & Luxon, 1998; Chery-Croze et al., 1993; Veuillet et al., 1991). A few patients showed an increase in emission amplitude under the suppression condition (Chery-Croze et al., 1993). Graham and Hazell (1994) found higher test-retest variability in the amount of transient OAE suppression obtained with contralateral broadband noise in subjects with tinnitus than in subjects without tinnitus.

OTOACOUSTIC EMISSIONS AND HEREDITARY HEARING LOSS

Understanding the factors underlying hereditary hearing loss is based on locating the genes responsible for hearing loss and defining the specific mechanisms and functions of those genes. From a clinical standpoint, understanding the characteristics of hereditary hearing loss and the impact of genetic factors on hearing may improve management strategies for individuals with hereditary hearing loss and their families. Accurate determination of the auditory characteristics associated with various genetic abnormalities requires the use of measures sensitive to subtle aspects of auditory function. Since most hereditary hearing losses are cochlear in origin, OAEs may be helpful in delineating hearing losses and contributing to the understanding of underlying mechanisms associated with genetic abnormalities.

Applications of OAEs in Hereditary Hearing Loss

Audiometric testing provides a baseline measure while other, more sensitive, measures (such as otoacoustic emissions, efferent reflexes, and auditory evoked potentials) are necessary to understand the nature of a hearing loss in more detail. Such detailed information regarding the characteristics of a hearing loss is important in understanding the relationship, or lack of relationship, between genotype and phenotype. (Note: Genotype describes an individual's genetic constitution. Phenotype relates to the physical characteristics of an individual and can include information obtained from physiological, morphological, and biochemical studies.) Because of their sensitivity to cochlear dysfunction, OAEs may be particularly well suited to clinical evaluation and research related to hereditary hearing loss.

Most hereditary hearing losses, since they are cochlear in nature, demonstrate abnormal OAEs (e.g., Borg , Samuelsson, & Dahl, 2000; Pak, Ng, Leung, & van Hasselt, 2000; Pfister et al., 1999). Several studies have demonstrated the sensitivity of otoacoustic emissions to auditory dysfunction in Waardenburg syndrome (Liu & Newton, 1997), Usher syndrome (Wagenaar, Snik, Kimberling, & Cremers, 1996), and in mitochondrial disorders (Sue et al., 1998), as well as in patients with nonsyndromic hearing loss (Lina-Granade, Collet, & Morgon, 1995). For example, Liu and Newton (1997) studied normally hearing patients with Waardenburg syndrome and noted that the majority of subjects showed notches in distortion product OAEs despite normal audiometric thresholds. In that study, the number of ears with abnormal OAEs (87.5%) was much higher than in normal control subjects (10%).

OAEs in Carriers of Genes for Hearing Loss

OAEs may also be helpful in understanding whether carriers of genes for hearing loss have subtle differences in auditory function. Individuals are heterozygous for a characteristic when they carry one normal and one abnormal copy of a particular gene. In recessive hereditary hearing loss, each parent carries one normal and one abnormal copy. Since two abnormal copies are necessary in recessive hearing loss to display the trait (in this case hearing loss), each parent must have one abnormal copy to contribute. Thus, while not displaying the trait, the parents are "obligate" carriers of the abnormal gene.

The majority of past studies of auditory function in obligate carriers of genes for hereditary hearing loss have used standard puretone audiometric thresholds, Bekesy audiometry, middle ear muscle reflex thresholds, auditory brainstem responses, and some other clinical behavioral audiologic tests to characterize hearing with mixed results. Some have reported differences in carrier from control subjects demonstrated by "dips" in the audiometric contour using Bekesy audiometry and a number of subjects with elevated middle ear muscle reflex thresholds (Anderson & Wedenberg, 1968, 1976). Another set of studies found no differences between obligate carriers of recessive deafness and control subjects (Eldridge, Berlin, Money, & McKusick,

1968; Konigsmark, Hollander, & Berlin, 1968; Mengel, Koningsmark, Berlin, & McKusick, 1967). The failure to find reliable audiologic abnormalities in normal hearing obligate carriers has been reiterated regularly in the literature (e.g., Cohen et al., 1996; Jaber et al., 1992; Konigsmark, 1971, 1972a, 1972b; Liu & Xu, 1994; Madell & Sculerati, 1991; Nance & McConnell, 1973; Oeken & Konig, 1993; Ruben & Rozycki, 1971; Taylor, Hine, Brasier, Chiveralls, & Morris, 1975). Techniques using microstructural audiometric analysis have shown presence of notches in obligate carriers of genes related to nonsyn-dromic recessive hearing loss (Stephens et al., 1995). Audiometric notches in the 500- to 3000-Hz frequency range were found using a computerized sweep frequency technique in carriers of recessive hear-ing loss associated with Usher syndrome (Meredith, Stephens, Sirimanna, Meyer-Bisch, & Reardon, 1992).

Otoacoustic emissions provide an opportunity to apply a meas-ure sensitive to cochlear integrity to this problem. We have observed that parents who are obligate carriers of the Acadian Usher syndrome type IC gene show decreased distortion product OAE amplitude in certain frequency areas (Hood, 1998; Hood et al., 2001), and that OAE amplitude is reduced in carriers of GJB2 (connexin 26) mutations in the Orthodox Jewish Ashkenazi population (Hood et al., 2001; Morell et al., 1998). These findings suggest that OAEs may provide insight into cochlear function in carriers of abnormal genes related to hearing loss and that auditory function differs in carriers.

SUMMARY

Otoacoustic emissions provide a powerful clinical tool in the evalua-tion of various types of hearing loss and in understanding normal cochlear processing. Their objectivity and the ability to record responses in patients of all ages further adds to clinical usefulness in newborn hearing screening and as an important clinical cross-check with other test findings. The presence of OAEs in inner hair cell and/or neural loss is complemented by the lack of efferent suppres-sion, which adds another potential clinical tool. OAEs also show promise as sensitive indicators of the effects of excessive noise and ototoxic drugs. The sensitivity of OAEs to subtle differences in cochlear function are further demonstrated by changes in OAEs in cer-tain populations of carriers of genes associated with hearing loss.

Acknowledgments: Preparation of this manuscript was supported by the National Institute of Health (NIH) NIDCD grant R01 DC03579 to Linda J. Hood. Research at Kresge Hearing Research Laboratory is supported the NIH National Institute on Deafness and Other Communication Disorders, U.S. Department of Defense, American Hearing Research Foundation, National Organization for Hearing Research, Deafness Research Foundation, Oberkotter Foundation, Kam's Fund for Hearing Research, Marriott Foundation, Kleberg Foundation, and the Louisiana Lions Eye Foundation. Contributions to cited research studies at Kresge Hearing Research Laboratory were made by the following individuals: Harriet Berlin, MA, Jill Bordelon, MCD, Shanda Brashears, MCD, Leah Goforth-Barter, MS, Annette Hurley, MS, Jennifer Jeanfreau, MCD, Bronya Keats, PhD, Elizabeth Montgomery, MS, Thierry Morlet, PhD, Kelly Rose, MA, Patti St. John, MA, Sonya Tedesco, MCD, Han Wen, MSBE, and Diane Wilensky, MA.

REFERENCES

Amatuzzi, M. G., Northrop, C., Liberman, M. C., Thornton, A., Halpin, C., Herrmann, B., Pinto, L. E., Saenz, A., Carranza, A., & Eavey, R. D. (2001). Selective inner hair cell loss in premature infants and cochlea pathological patterns from neonatal intensive care unit autopsies. *Archives of Otolaryngology-Head Neck Surgery, 127*, 629–636.

Anderson, H., & Wedenberg, E. (1968). Audiometric identification of normal hearing carriers of genes for deafness. *Acta Oto-laryngologica, 65*, 535–554.

Anderson, H., & Wedenberg, E. (1976). Identification of normal hearing carriers of genes for deafness. *Acta Oto-laryngologica, 83*, 245–248.

Berlin, C. I., Bordelon, J., St. John, P., Wilensky, D., Hurley, A., Kluka, E., & Hood, L. J. (1998). Reversing click polarity may uncover auditory neuropathy in infants. *Ear and Hearing, 19*, 37–47.

Berlin, C. I., Hood, L. J., Cecola, R. P., Jackson, D. F., & Szabo P. (1993). Does type I afferent neuron dysfunction reveal itself through lack of efferent suppression? *Hearing Research, 65*, 40–50.

Berlin, C. I., Hood, L. J., Hurley, A., & Wen, H. (1994). Contralateral suppression of otoacoustic emissions: An index of the function of the medial olivocochlear system. *Otolaryngology-Head Neck Surgery, 100*, 3–21.

Berlin, C. I., Hood, L. J., Hurley, A., Wen, H., & Kemp, D. T. (1995). Bilateral noise suppresses click-evoked otoacoustic emissions more than ipsilateral or contralateral noise. *Hearing Research, 87*, 96–103.

Berlin, C. I., Hood, L. J., Goforth-Barter, L., & Bordelon, J. (1999). Clinical applications of auditory efferent studies. In C. I. Berlin (Ed.). *The efferent auditory system* (pp. 105–124). San Diego, CA: Singular Publishing Group.

Berlin, C. I., Hood, L. J., Wen, H., Szabo, P., Cecola, R. P., Rigby, P., & Jackson, D. F. (1993). Contralateral suppression of non-linear click-evoked otoacoustic emissions. *Hearing Research, 71*, 1–11.

Berlin, C. I., Szabo, P., Cecola, P., Hood. L, J., Rigby, P., Erato, R., Fontenot, C., & Allen, J. (1991). Comparison of evoked otoacoustic emissions and distortion product emissions via the Kemp and cubic distortion product systems. *ARO Abstracts, 14,* 66.

Borg, E., Samuelsson, E., & Dahl, N. (2000).Audiometric characterization of a family with digenic autosomal, dominant, progressive sensorineural hearing loss. *Oto-laryngologica, 120,* 51–57.

Brownell, W. E, Bader, C. R., Bertrand D., & de Ribaupierre, Y. (1985). Evoked mechanical responses of isolated cochlear outer hair cells. *Science, 227,* 194–196.

Castor, X., Veuillet, E., Morgon, A., & Collet, L. (1994). Influence of aging on active cochlear micromechanical properties and on the medial olivo-cochlear system in humans. *Hearing Research, 77,* 1–8.

Ceranic, B. J., Prasher, D. K., Raglan, E., & Luxon, L. M. (1998). Tinnitus after head injury: Evidence from otoacoustic emissions. *Journal of Neurology, Neurosurgery & Psychiatry, 65,* 523–529.

Chery-Croze, S., Collet, L., & Morgon, A. (1993). Medial olivo-cochlear system and tinnitus. *Acta Oto-laryngologica (Stockholm), 113,* 285–290.

Cohen, M., Francis, M., Luxon, L. M., Bellman, S., Coffey, R., & Pembrey, M. (1996). Dips on Bekesy or Audioscan fail to identify carriers of autosomal recessive non-syndromic hearing loss. *Acta Oto-laryngologica (Stockholm), 116,* 521–527.

Collet, L., Kemp, D. T., Veuillet, E., Duclaux, R., Moulin, A., & Morgon, A. (1990). Effect of contralateral auditory stimuli on active cochlear micro-mechanical properties in human subjects. *Hearing Research, 43,* 251–262.

Eldridge, R., Berlin, C. I., Money, J. W., & McKusick, V. A. (1968). Cochlear deafness, myopia, and intellectual impairment in an Amish family. *Archives of Otolaryngology-Head Neck Surgery, 88,* 75–80.

Engdahl, B., Arnensen, A. R., & Mair, I. W. S. (1994). Reproducibility and short-term variation of transient evoked otoacoustic emissions. *Scandinavian Audiology, 23,* 99–104.

Giraud, A. L., Collet, L., Chery-Croze, S., Magnan, J., & Chays, A. (1995). Evidence of a medial olivocochlear involvement in contralateral suppression of otoacoustic emissions in humans. *Brain Research, 705,* 15–23.

Glattke, T. J., & Kujawa, S. G. (1991). Otoacoustic emissions. *American Journal of Audiology, 1,* 29-40.

Goforth, L., Hood, L., Morlet, T., Li, L., Reddy, S., & Berlin, C. (2000). Update on the development of neonatal efferent auditory function. *ARO Abstracts, 23,* 159.

Graham, R. L., & Hazell, J. W. (1994). Contralateral suppression of transient evoked otoacoustic emissions: Intra-individual variability in tinnitus and normal subjects. *British Journal of Audiology, 28,* 235–245.

Hildesheimer, M., Hamburger, A., Ari-Even Roth, D., Muchnik, C., & Kuint, J. (1999). The maturation of the auditory efferent system in neonates tested by the suppression effect of transient evoked otoacoustic emission (TEOAE). *IERASG Abstracts, XVI,* VI–5.

Hood L. J. (1998). The role of otoacoustic emissions in identifying carriers of hereditary hearing loss. In C. I. Berlin (Ed.), *Otoacoustic emissions. Basic science and clinical applications* (pp. 137–148). San Diego, CA: Singular Publishing Group.

Hood, L. J., Berlin, C. I., Bordelon, J., Goforth-Barter, L., Hurley, A., & Tedesco, S. (2000). Patients with auditory neuropathy lack efferent suppression of transient evoked otoacoustic emissions. *ARO Abstracts, 23,* 159.

Hood, L. J., Berlin, C. I., Goforth-Barter, L., Bordelon, J., Wen, H. (1999). Recording and analyzing efferent suppression of transient-evoked otoacoustic emissions. In C. I. Berlin (Ed.), *The efferent auditory system.* San Diego, CA: Singular Publishing Group.

Hood, L. J., Berlin, C. I., Hurley, A., Cecola, R. P., & Bell, B. (1996). Contralateral suppression of click-evoked otoacoustic emissions: Intensity effects. *Hearing Research, 101,* 113–118.

Hood, L. J., Hurley, A. E., Goforth, L., Bordelon, J., & Berlin, C. I. (1997). Aging and efferent suppression of otoacoustic emissions. *ARO Abstracts, 20,* 167.

Hood, L. J., Berlin, C. I., Tedesco, S., Brashears, S., Jeanfreau, J., Keats, B. J., & Morlet, T. (2001). Otoacoustic emissions in carriers of genes for hearing loss. *ARO Abstracts, 24,* 267.

Jaber, L., Shohat, M., Bu, X., Fischel-Ghodsian, N., Yang, H. Y., Wang, S. J., & Rotler, J. I. (1992). Sensorineural deafness inherited as a tissue specific mitochondrial disorder. *Journal of Medical Genetics, 29,* 86–90.

Kemp, D. T. (1978). Stimulated acoustic emissions from within the human auditory system. *Journal of the Acoustical Society of America, 64,* 1386–1391.

Kemp, D. T., & Chum, R. (1980). Properties of the generator of stimulated acoustic emissions. *Hearing Research, 2,* 213–232.

Khanna, S. M., & Leonard, D. G. (1982). Basilar membrane tuning in the cat cochlea. *Science, 215,* 305–306.

Konigsmark, B. W. (1971). Hereditary congenital severe deafness syndromes. *Annals of Otolology, Rhinology, and Laryngology, 80,* 269–288.

Konigsmark, B. W. (1972a). Genetic hearing loss with no associated abnormalities: A review. *The Journal of Speech and Hearing Disorders, 37,* 89–99.

Konigsmark, B. W. (1972b). Hereditary childhood hearing loss and integumentary system disease. *The Journal of Pediatrics, 80,* 909–919.

Konigsmark, B. W., Hollander, M. B., & Berlin, C. I. (1968). Familial neural hearing loss and atopic dermatitis. *Journal of the American Medical Association, 204,* 953–957.

Liang, F., Liu, C., & Liu, B. (1997). Otoacoustic emission and auditory efferent function testing in patients with sensori-neural hearing loss. *Chinese Medical Journal, 110,* 139–141.

Liberman, M. C., & Guinan, J. J., Jr. (1998). Feedback control of the auditory periphery: Anti-masking effects of middle ear muscles vs. olivocochlear efferents. *Journal of Communication Disorders, 31,* 471–482.

Lina-Granade, G., Collet, L., & Morgon, A. (1995). Physiopathological investigations in a family with a history of unilateral hereditary deafness. *Acta Oto-laryngologica, 115,* 196–201.

Liu, X. Z., & Newton, V. E. (1997). Distortion product emissions in normal-hearing and low-frequency hearing loss carriers of genes for Waardenburg's syndrome. *Annals of Otolology, Rhinology, and Laryngology, 106*, 220–225.

Liu, X., & Xu, L. (1994). Nonsyndromic hearing loss: An analysis of audio-grams. *Annals of Otolology, Rhinology, and Laryngology, 103*, 428–433.

Madell, J. R., & Sculerati, N. (1991). Noncongenital hereditary hearing loss in children. *Archives of Otolaryngology-Head Neck Surgery, 117*, 332–335.

Martin, G. K., Probst, R., Lonsbury-Martin, B. L. (1990). Otoacoustic emissions in human ears: Normative findings. *Ear & Hearing, 11*, 106–120.

Maurer, J., Beck, W., Mann, W., & Mintert, R. (1992). Veränderungen otoakustischer Emissionen unto gleichzeitiger Beschallung des Gegenohres bei Normalpersonen und bei Patientien mit einseitigem Akustikusneurinom. [Changes of amplitude of otoacoustic emissions under contralateral noise in normal hearing persons and in patients with unilateral acoustic neuroma.] *Laryngology-Rhinology-Otology, 71*, 69–73.

Mengel, M. C., Konigsmark B. W., Berlin, C. I., & McKusick, V. A. (1967). Recessive early-onset neural deafness. *Acta Oto-laryngologica, 64*, 313–326.

Meredith, R., Stephens, D., Sirimanna, T., Meyer-Bisch, C., & Reardon, W. (1992). Audiometric detection of carriers of Usher's syndrome type II. *Journal of Audiologic Medicine, 1*, 11–19.

Micheyl, C., Carbonnel, O., & Collet, L. (1995). Medial olivocochlear system and loudness adaptation: Differences between musicians and non-musicians. *Brain Cognition, 29*, 127–136.

Micheyl, C., Morlet, T., Giraud, A. L., Collet, L., & Morgon, A. (1995a). Contralateral suppression of evoked otoacoustic emissions and detection of a multi-tone complex in noise. *Acta Oto-laryngologica, 115*, 178–182.

Morell, R. J., Kim, H. J., Hood, L. J., Goforth, L., Friderici, K., Fisher, R., Van Camp, G., Berlin, C. I., Oddoux, C., Ostrer, H., Keats, B., & Friedman, T. B. (1998). Mutations in the connexin 26 gene (GJB2) among Ashkenazi Jews with nonsyndromic recessive deafness. *New England Journal of Medicine, 339*, 1500–1505.

Morlet, T., Collet, L., Salle, B., & Morgon, A. (1993). Functional maturation of cochlear active mechanisms and of the medial olivocochlear system in humans. *Acta Otolaryngologica (Stockholm), 113*, 271–277.

Morlet, T., Goforth, L., Hood, L. J., Ferber, C., Duclaux, R., & Berlin, C. I. (1999). Development of human cochlear active mechanism asymmetry: Involvement of the medial olivocochlear system? *Hearing Research, 134*, 153–162.

Mott, J. B., Norton, S. J., Neely, S. T., & Warr, W. B. (1989). Changes in spontaneous otoacoustic emissions produced by acoustic stimulation of the contralateral ear. *Hearing Research, 38*, 229–242.

Moulin, A., Collet, L., & Duclaux, R. (1993). Contralateral auditory stimulation alters acoustic distortion products in humans. *Hearing Research, 65*, 193–210.

Moulin, A., Collet, L., & Morgon, A. (1992). Influence of spontaneous otoacoustic emissions (SOAE) on acoustic distortion product input/output functions: Does the medial efferent system act differently in the vicinity of an SOAE? *Acta Oto-laryngologica, 112,* 210–4.

Nance, W. E., & McConnell, F. E. (1973). Status and prospects of research in hereditary deafness. In H. Harris & K. Hirschorn (Eds.), *Advances in human genetics* (Vol. 4, pp. 175–250). New York: Plenum Press.

Nieschall, M., Beneking, R., & Stoll, W. (1997). Increased amplitude of distortion product emissions in the human caused by contralateral low intensity acoustic stimulation. *HNO, 45,* 378–384.

Oeken, J., & Konig, E. (1993). Forms of monosymptomatic hereditary sensorineural hearing loss and deafness in the Leipzig area. *HNO, 41,* 301–310.

Ohlms, L. A., Lonsbury-Martin, B. L., & Martin, G. K. (1990). The clinical application of acoustic distortion products. *Otolaryngology-Head Neck Surgery, 103,* 52–59.

Pak, M. W., Ng, M. H., Leung, C. B., & van Hasselt, C. A. (2000). Cochlear deafness in a Chinese family with Fechtner's syndrome. *American Journal of Otology, 21,* 345–350.

Pfister, M. H., Apaydin, F., Turan, O., Bereketoglu, M., Bilgen, V., Braendle, U., Kose, S., Zenner, H. P., & Lalwani, A. K. (1999). Clinical evidence for dystrophin dysfunction as a cause of hearing loss in locus DFN4. *Laryngoscope, 109,* 730–735.

Prasher, D., Ryan, S., & Luxon, L. (1994). Contralateral suppression of transiently evoked otoacoustic emission and neuro-otology. *British Journal of Audiology, 28,* 247–254.

Prasher, D. K., Tun, T., Brookes, G. B., & Luxon, L. M. (1995). Mechanisms of hearing loss in acoustic neuroma: An otoacoustic emission study. *Acta Otolaryngologica (Stockholm), 115,* 375–381.

Probst, R., Lonsbury-Martin, B. L., & Martin, G. K. (1991). A review of otoacoustic emissions. *Journal of the Acoustical Society of America, 89,* 2027–2067.

Rabinowitz, W. M., & Widen, G. P. (1984). Interaction of spontaneous otoacoustic emissions and external sounds. *Journal of the Acoustical Society of America, 76,* 1713–1720.

Robinette, M. S., & Durrant, J. D. (1997). Contributions of evoked otoacoustic emissions in differential diagnosis of retrocochlear lesions. In M. S. Robinette & T. J. Glattke (Eds.). *Otoacoustic emissions: Clinical applications* (pp. 205–232). New York: Thieme.

Roede, J., Harris, F. P., Probst, R., & Xu, L. (1993). Repeatability of distortion product otoacoustic emissions in normally hearing humans. *Audiology, 32,* 273–281.

Ruben, R. J., & Rozycki, D. L. (1971). Clinical aspects of genetic deafness. *Annals of Otology, Rhinology, and Laryngology, 80,* 255–263.

Ryan, S., & Kemp, D. T. (1996). The influence of evoking stimulus level on the neural suppression of transient evoked otoacoustic emissions. *Hearing Research, 94,* 140–147.

Ryan, S., Kemp, D. T., & Hinchcliffe, R. (1991). The influence of contralateral acoustic stimulation on click-evoked otoacoustic emissions in humans. *British Journal of Audiology, 25,* 391–397.

Ryan, S., & Piron, J. P. (1994). Functional maturation of the medial olivo-cochlear system in human neonates. *Acta Otolaryngologica (Stockholm), 144,* 485–489.

Schloth, E., & Zwicker, E. (1983). Mechanical and acoustic influences on spontaneous otoacoustic emission. *Hearing Research, 11,* 285–293.

Starr, A., McPherson, D., Patterson, J., Don, M., Luxford, W., Shannon, R., Sininger, Y., Tonokawa, L., & Waring, M. (1991). Absence of both auditory evoked potentials and auditory percepts depending on timing cues. *Brain, 114,* 1157–1180.

Starr, A., Picton, T. W., Sininger, Y., Hood, L. J., & Berlin, C. I. (1996). Auditory neuropathy. *Brain, 119,* 741–753.

Stephens, D., Meredith, R., Sirimanna, T., France, L., Almqvist, C., & Haugen, H. (1995). Application of the audioscan in the detection of carriers of genetic hearing loss. *Audiology, 34,* 91–97.

Sue, C. M., Lipsett L. J., Crimmins, D. S., Tsang, C. S., Boyages, S. C., Presgrave, C. M., Gibson, W. P., Byrne, E., & Morris, J. G. (1998). Cochlear origin of hearing loss in MELAS syndrome. *Annals of Neurology, 43,* 350–359.

Taylor, I. G., Hine, W. D., Brasier, V. J., Chiveralls, K., & Morris, T. (1975). A study of the causes of hearing loss in a population with special reference to genetic factors. *The Journal of Laryngology and Otology, 89,* 899–914.

Timpe-Syverson, G. K., & Decker, T. N. (1999). Attention effects on distortion-product otoacoustic emissions with contralateral speech stimuli. *Journal of the American Academy of Audiology, 10,* 371–378.

Veuillet, E., Collet, L., & Duclaux, R. (1991). Effect of contralateral acoustic stimulation on active cochlear micromechanical properties in human subjects: Dependence on stimulus variables. *Journal of Neurophysiology, 65,* 724–735.

Wagenaar, M., Snik, A. F., Kimberling, W. J., & Cremers, C. W. (1996). Carriers of the Usher syndrome type IB: Is audiometric identification possible? *American Journal of Otology, 17,* 853–858.

Warr, W. B., & Guinan, J. J. (1978). Efferent innervation of the organ of Corti: Two different systems. *Brain Research, 173,* 152–155.

Warr, W. B., Guinan, J. J., & White, J. S. (1986). Organization of the efferent fibers: The lateral and medial olivocochlear systems. In R. A. Altschuler, R. P. Bobbin, & D. W. Hoffman (Eds.). *Neurobiology of hearing: The cochlea* (pp. 333–348). New York: Raven Press.

Wen, H., Berlin, C. I., Hood, L. J., Jackson, D., & Hurley, A. (1993). A program for the quantification and analysis of transient evoked otoacoustic emissions. *ARO Abstracts, 16,* 102.

Williams, E. A., Brookes, G. B., & Prasher, D. K. (1993). Effects of contralateral acoustic stimulation on otoacoustic emissions following vestibular neurectomy. *Scandinavian Audiology, 22,* 197–203.

Williams, E. A., Brookes, G. B., & Prasher, D. K. (1994). Effects of olivocochlear bundle section on otoacoustic emissions in humans: Efferent effects in comparison with control subjects. *Acta Otolaryngologica, 114,* 121–129.

8

The Physiological Bases of Audiological Management

Charles I. Berlin, PhD
Linda J. Hood, PhD
Jennifer Jeanfreau, MCD
Thierry Morlet, PhD
Shanda Brashears, MCD
Department of Otolaryngology

Bronya Keats, PhD
Department of Otolaryngology and Genetics
Louisiana State University Health Sciences Center
New Orleans, Louisiana

INTRODUCTION

The chapters in this book are unique in that they sweep from microstructural and molecular mechanisms, through genetic under-pinnings of deafness, to efferent function. It falls to us to bring a unifying set of principles that are clinically useful. We will try to outline a straightforward plan buttressed by a logical rationale. The first set of recommendations applies to newborns and infants, but is in part applicable to adults.

The message is that, as of today, every new patient in whom a definitive audiological diagnosis is sought should be tested with the following procedures, which we will call the Triage Trio:

1. Tympanometry (at 660 Hz or higher if an infant)
2. Middle ear muscle reflexes
3. Otoacoustic emissions

Depending on the results of these three tests, various diagnostic strategies might be invoked that in turn may shed light on proper management. These three tests can generate six possible combinations of results, each of which points to a different set of diagnostic and management categories. However, one result, *normal emissions and absent middle ear muscle reflexes*, suggests that both any subsequent routine monopolar or alternating polarity auditory brainstem response (ABR) and any behavioral audiograms may lead to incorrect management. In such cases, an ABR with one positive and one negative polarity click is needed, not to assess hearing but to assess neural synchrony (Berlin et al., 1998). If the ABR is abnormal or absent, but emissions are present, hearing aids are not usually appropriate, while cochlear implants may work quite well if the child does not spontaneously outgrow the problem. See Table 8–1 later in the chapter.

The big picture, according to "old wisdom," suggested that there are basically two types of organic peripheral hearing loss: conductive and sensorineural. "Old wisdom" taught that the former are treatable by medicine or surgery, but the latter is not treatable medically at all and calls for hearing aids with no great expectations as to results. The diagnostic categories were built on tuning fork test results and audiologic evaluations by air conduction and bone conduction.

It is clear that the mammalian ear is one of the most complicated sense organs in nature, with over 100,000 moving parts. We will show you how there might be at least 70 different ways in which cochlear hearing loss can occur, some of which are treatable both medically and surgically. It naturally follows that many different conditions of the inner ear can lead to similar audiograms, which, when interpreted through the audiologic context of tympanometry, reflexes, and emissions, might lead to vastly different managements. At the end of this chapter we will show four patients with severe deafness by pure tone audiometry, whose tympanometry, reflexes, and emissions all suggest different underlying physiologic conditions of the cochlea and hair cells. Thus, it is useful to inject a brief review of cochlear physiology and show why this Triage Trio, at least in terms of today's audiology, is so useful.

THE FIVE ELECTROACOUSTIC EVENTS IN THE COCHLEA

Endocochlear Potential (EP)

The endocochlear potential (EP) is the 80–100 +mv battery that drives virtually all the clinically measurable effects in the human cochlea. Figure 8–1 shows that the potential is made up of the algebraic sum of a +140 mv aerobic potential and a –60 mv anaerobic potential.

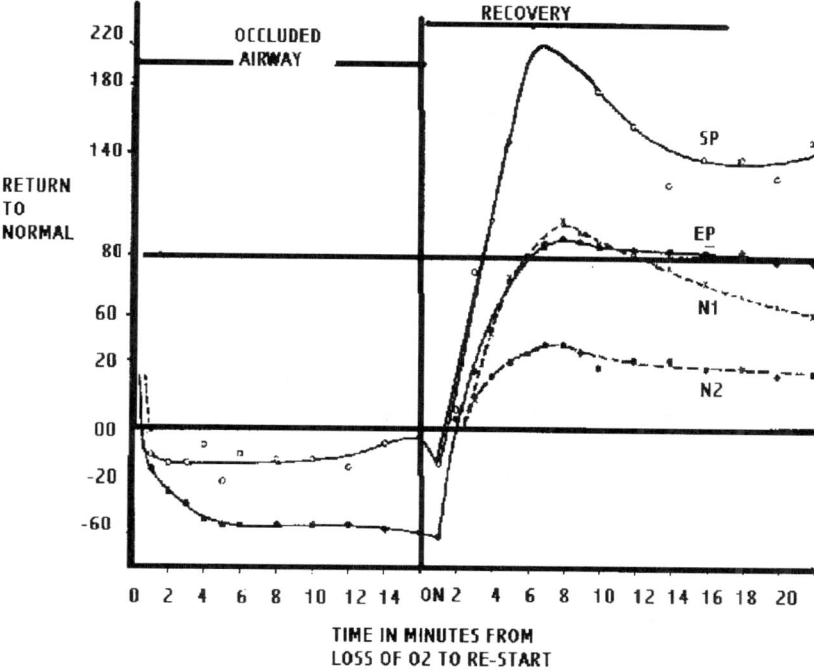

Figure 8–1. Time course of the endocochlear potential after airway is occluded. From Konishi et al. (1961).

Figure 8–1 also shows how all the other potentials of the inner ear change drastically when the EP is affected by oxygen deprivation.

The EP is the only one of these five events that is *not* currently measurable in humans. When we become able to measure this potential clinically, many new inner ear conditions will become clarified.

At present, while this potential is not directly measurable in humans, its presence can be inferred when otoacoustic emissions and cochlear microphonics are present. Thus, one of the first advantages of observing a cochlear microphonic and/or otoacoustic emissions is a confirmation of the integrity of the stria vascularis and Reissner's membrane, whose collective integrity is probably required for the maintenance of the endochlear potential.

Cochlear Microphonic

The cochlear microphonic (CM), or cochlear potential, was first reported by Wever and Bray in 1930 (Wever, 1959). At the time the authors recorded it as part of their electrical study of the inner ear and properly named it cochlear potential. However, some of their contemporaries thought it was an epiphenomenon and gave it the somewhat derogatory appellation of "microphonic," suggesting it was irrelevant to important cochlear activity.

What we now know is that the CM reflects the presence of, and electrical field surrounding, both outer and inner hair cells. In humans, its presence usually signifies primarily, but not only, outer hair cell activity at the basal turn. One of its salient characteristics, about which we shall talk in greater detail later, is that it is polarity sensitive. That is to say, when the polarity of the stimulus used to elicit it is inverted, the electrical recording also inverts. (See the CD in this volume.)

This particular characteristic of the CM will have great significance in the proper interpretation of diagnostic auditory brainstem responses (ABRs), as we shall see later.

Compound Action Potential

The compound action potential (CAP or N_1N_2) represents the synchronous depolarization/discharge of many single units of the auditory nerve. It is best visualized using a brief stimulus that synchronously discharges many units from the basal turn within a couple of milliseconds. Units from the more apical regions of the cochlea are discharged in a less synchronized fashion, consistent with traveling wave delays and mechanics. See Kemp's CD-ROM (1998) for interactive computer simulations of traveling wave micromechanics where the reader can choose the frequency of stimulation and watch the basilar membrane model change its mechanical motion. The simulation can show active cochlear mechanics and distortion products if so desired.

One of its salient characteristics is that the averaged waveform representing the CAP does *not* invert with polarity of the stimulus, but instead changes its latency only by one half period of the stimulation cycle (Figure 8–2).

It is certainly possible, if not common, to have a cochlear microphonic recordable without otoacoustic emissions being recordable (Withnell, 2001).

Thus, we can see that to separate hair cell function and cochlear microphonic from neural function and the CAP, one need only invert the polarity of the stimulus to properly differentiate the responses that may occupy overlapping time periods after stimulation.

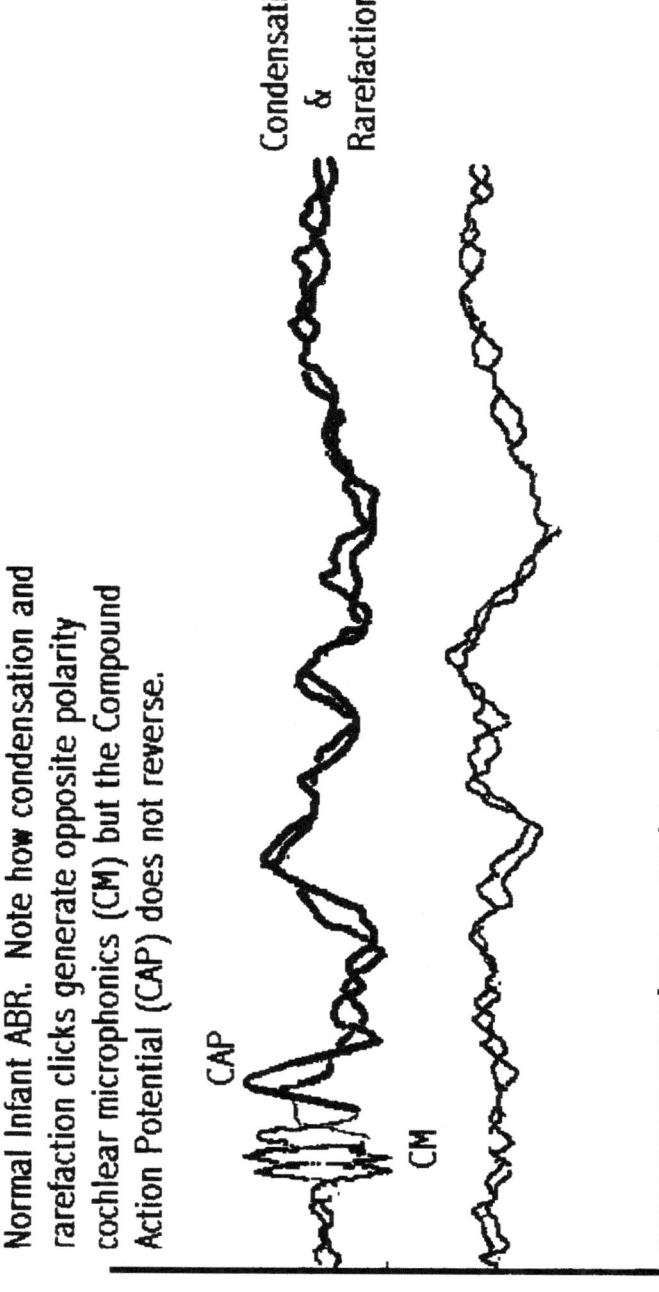

Figure 8–2. A normal infant's ABR including an inverting cochlear microphonic at the beginning and CAP and normal waveforms thereafter.

143

Summating Potential

The summating potential (SP) is a DC offset potential of the CM, which lasts for the duration of the stimulus. When the stimulus is a long tone burst, the SP follows the envelope of that tone burst (see Figure 8–3). If the stimulus were a brief click, the SP would briefly shift off the baseline in either positive or negative direction. Its amplitude relative to CAP is considered diagnostic for cochlear hydrops (Eggermont & Odenthal, 1974).

The source of the summating potential is in some doubt, some ascribing it to outer hair cells (OHCs), others to inner hair cells (IHCs) (Cheatham & Dallos, 1984), and others to both (Durrant, Wang, Ding, & Salvi, 1998). In auditory dys-synchrony patients, in whom we presume have primarily OHC function, the SP can sometimes be observed. However, it is not yet clear why the SP is present in some patients and not in others.

Otoacoustic Emissions (OAEs)

Otoacoustic emissions (OHC), first described by Kemp (1978) after others had erroneously ascribed the spontaneous variety to vascular or muscular noises, are sounds that come from the cochlea. The consensus is that they arise from outer hair cells in mammals, even if they are seen in species that do not have outer and inner hair cells differentiated. There are four different types of emissions that are currently recognizable: spontaneous (see above), transient evoked, distortion product (with a number of subcategories), and stimulus evoked. Although "current wisdom" implies that emissions arise from the micromechanics surrounding hair cells, there are suggestions that transient and distortion product emissions represent different mechanisms of the process (Shera & Guinan, 1999). When we see emissions in a human patient, we can be assured that the endocochlear potential, the OHCs, and the middle ear (which allows passage of the faint sounds) are all reasonably normal.

This inference is extremely powerful, since it tells us that four of the five electroacoustic potentials in the inner ear are functional, and that we should see a robust CAP and vigorous middle ear reflex contractions in response to an intense brief stimulus.

It is precisely because this physiologic information is revealed by the presence of emissions and middle ear reflexes that we recommend to our audiological colleagues that these three tests be mandatory in any new diagnostic patient.

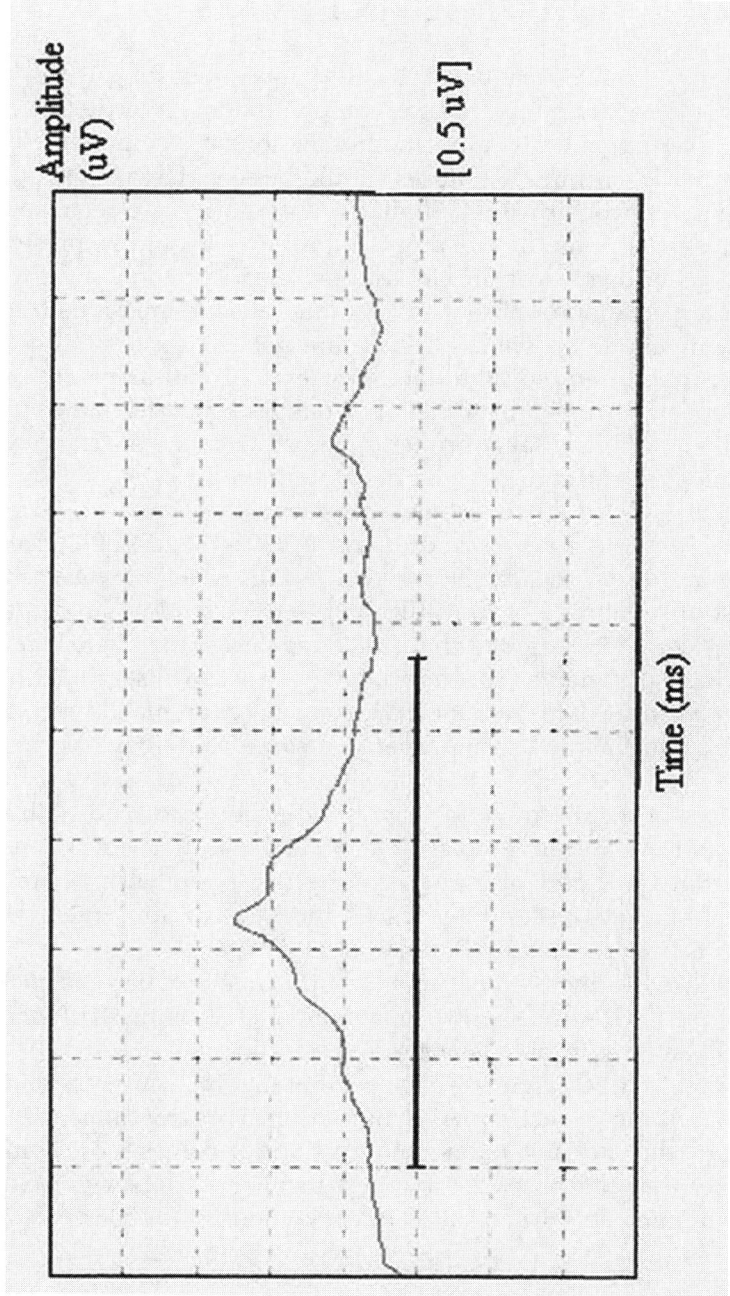

Figure 8–3. A summating potential recorded with a 14 msec 2 kHz tone. Time scale 3 msec/div.

HOW THEY INTERACT AND ARE
INTERPRETED IN HUMANS

We have urged our colleagues to begin diagnostic testing with three procedures: tympanometry, reflexes, and emissions. Interpretation of the tests is contingent one upon another. As long as tympanometry is normal, middle ear muscle reflexes should be seen. Unless, of course, there is a severe cochlear loss. Similarly, if emissions are seen, severe hearing loss is supposedly ruled out and reflexes should be present if there is no conductive loss. Again, to show the interaction of the tests, proper interpretation of absent reflexes and absent emissions hinges on the tympanometry. Thus, all three are needed almost at once in order to properly employ the data. However, if emissions are seen, tympanometry can be presumed normal and middle ear muscle reflexes then become vital to proper diagnosis. Hence a special plea to my audiological colleagues . . . do not skip the reflexes!

Table 8–1 shows some sample outcomes.

If the patient is a newborn or infant, ABR is the test of choice for assessing auditory function. However, the ABR is *not a test of hearing*, but a test of synchrony of the VIIIth nerve fibers and auditory pathways. It is commonly agreed that IHCs depolarize the afferent nerve fibers of the VIIIth nerve (Spoendlin, 1985). Thus, an absent ABR need not mean cochlear damage but could mean either an inability to stimulate IHCs and their neurons properly or some pathology of primary neurons.

Therefore, we recommend that the ABR be performed with one positive and one negative polarity click, to separate cochlear microphonic from CAP and properly discriminate neural from hair cell function. In Figures 8–4 and 8–5 we see the value of this strategy, had the subjects been newborns (Berlin et al., 1998).

In Figure 8–6 the cochlear microphonic inverts when the click is inverted, the CAP shifts slightly in latency, and the entire ABR shows an orderly and predictable latency-intensity function.

In stark contrast, Figure 8–5 shows that the five waves elicited by the first click are in fact *not* ABR but cochlear microphonic. This is revealed by the click inversion maneuver and becomes more evident when one sees the absence of a lengthening of latencies with a decrease in intensity (the so-called latency-intensity function).

Table 8–1

Results	Diagnostic Likelihood
Tymps normal Reflexes present and symmetrical at 75–95 both ipsilaterally and contralaterally. Emissions present	Normal peripheral cochlear and brainstem function. Does not rule out upper brainstem or cortical deafness. Expect pure tone audiometry in the normal range by the time the child can be tested.
Tymps normal Reflexes present or sometimes elevated. Emissions absent at some or all frequencies.	Cochlear hearing loss. Expect audiogram to reflect peripheral hearing loss. Outer hair cell loss primarily. Expect normal ABR intervals and latencies. Robust Wave I at high intensities. Hearing aids usually help.
Tymps normal Reflexes absent Emissions present	This is the cardinal sign of auditory dys-synchrony/auditory neuropathy and requires an ABR be done with positive and negative polarity clicks to outline the cochlear microphonic and separate hair cell from neural function. When outer hair cells are normal in the entire frequency range, hearing aids are not usually useful. See later for management suggestions.
Tymps normal Reflexes absent Emissions absent	Expect severe to profound inner ear loss (but occasionally otosclerosis without affecting the tympanogram markedly).
Tymps abnormal Reflexes absent Emissions absent	Expect conductive or mixed loss but may also be severely deafened. Inner ear deafness is no inoculation against middle ear disease.

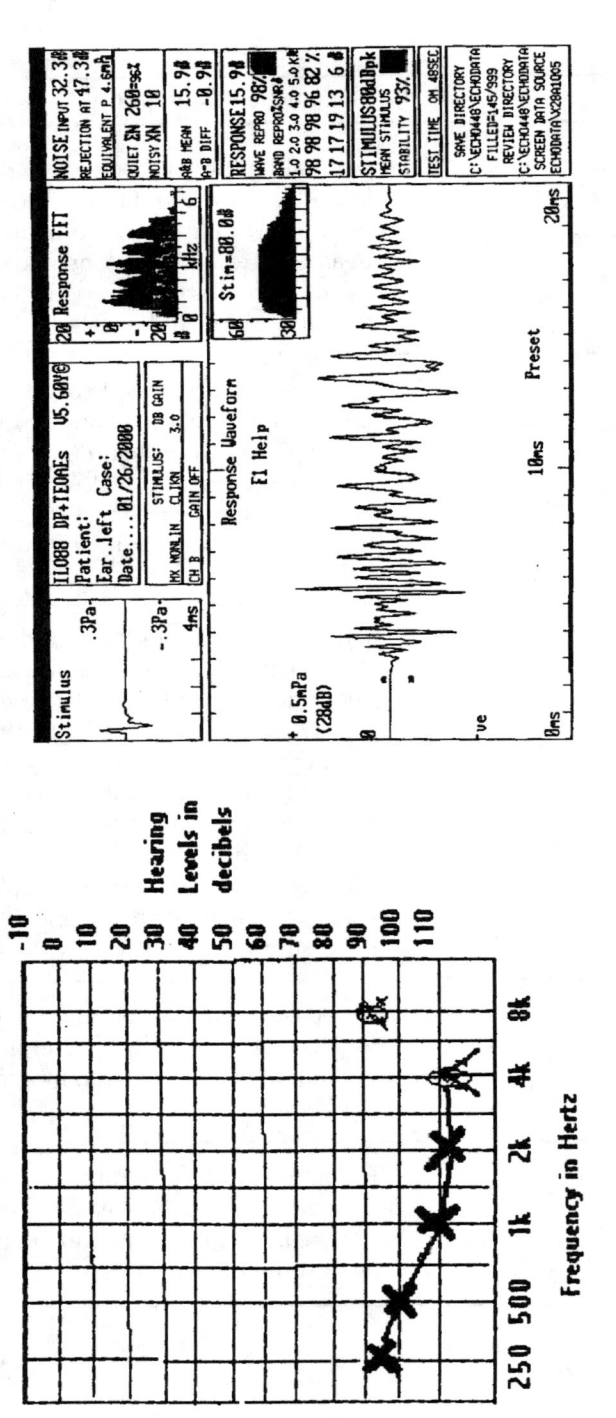

Behavioral Audiogram   Click Evoked Otoacoustic Emissions

Figure 8–4. Normal emissions in the presence of "pure tone deafness".

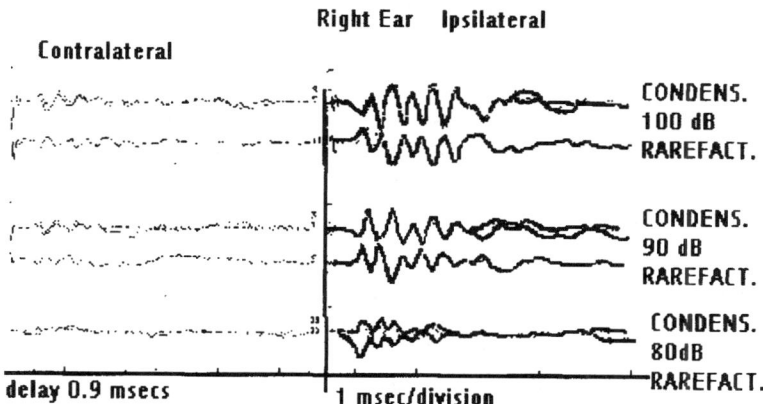

Figure 8–5. A totally inverting cochlear microphonic, which masquerades as an ABR until inverting clicks are used.

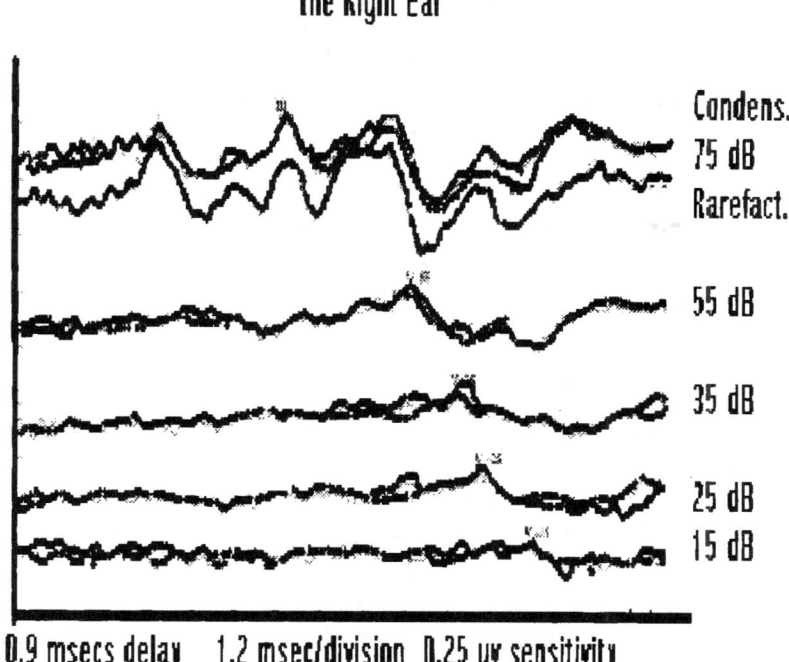

Figure 8–6. Normal latency-intensity function for a right ear.

HOW MANAGEMENT DERIVES FROM PHYSIOLOGY

Since the thesis of this chapter is that identical audiograms can be produced from vastly different physiological states, let us examine four examples representing six patients with identical so-called "corner audiograms." Because all the behavioral audiograms are virtually the same, only one need be shown.

Patient 1 and His Brother

This patient was referred by his parents and pediatrician for failure to develop speech and language. His diagnosis and management were consistent with a Scheibe deafness of a genetic nature. Genetic studies showed a connexin 26 deafness with a 35 del G mutation.

He had a normal birth at 40 weeks gestation and began to walk at 11 months, but did not babble canonically by even 1 year (Eilers & Berlin, 1995). He had a flat ABR, absent reflexes, and was observed to be behaviorally hearing impaired from his very first evaluation. He was aided by 1 year of age. Two-and-a-half years later his brother was born, and his mother called from the hospital certain that her second child was deaf as well. An ABR was completed at 1 week of age and repeated again at 3 weeks. His reflexes were absent and emissions were not available at the time. They have since been done and found to be absent. Both he and his brother did well in hearing aids and auditory verbal therapy, but reached a plateau with hearing aids and audition alone at about age 4½ for the older child and age 2 for the younger child. They have both since had cochlear implantation, with the younger child being the more successful auditorily and with both spoken language and speech clarity.

Patient 2 and Her Brother

This young girl was correctly observed by her parents to be unresponsive to sound.

She had a flat ABR and was behaviorally quite deaf. Her audiologists, however, elected to check otoacoustic emissions and were surprised to find them present. See Figure 8–4.

Both the family and the audiologists were taken aback and consulted us at this point because her audiologists knew we had recently reported seeing patients with absent ABRs and normal emissions. The family also had a second child, a boy, who presented with the same symptomatology. The parents elected cued speech as a communication method with both children and were quite successful at teaching them language, but they produced little intelligible speech. Therefore, they elected to attend an auditory verbal school in the hopes of having their children learn and communicate auditorily.

The leaders of this school felt they had to try hearing aids, but were also sophisticated enough to know that with normal OHC function, hearing aids might not do much more than increase sensitivity (Berlin, Hood, Hurley, & Wen, 1996). Therefore, they agreed to try just one hearing aid on the older child first and monitor emissions daily in both ears, since the child's normal emissions might involute with or without the trauma of amplification. The hearing aid was unsuccessful at eliciting spoken language and auditory behavior, so the parents elected to try cochlear implantation, first on their older child who had excellent language skills.

Reportedly, within a few days of the implant being activated, the child responded to a telephone ringing, picked it up, and identified her grandmother as the speaker. Four years later she is mainstreamed in a regular public school, is reading at the top of her class, and apparently needs no additional services. According to her parents, the child's excellent language and phonologic skills are traceable in large part to her early use of cued speech (Cornett & Daisy, 1992).

With the great auditory and speech success of their older child, the parents quickly elected cochlear implantation for their second child, who made similar progress auditorily, but because of a speech apraxia, was slower to speak than his sister. Both were among the first children with auditory neuropathy to be knowingly and successfully implanted.

In contrast to patient 1 and his brother, where auditory verbal methods and hearing aids were successful, patient 2 and her brother show that proper classification using otoacoustic emissions first pointed the family and audiologists away from auditory verbal methods and toward more visual representations of language. Once cochlear implantation was chosen, auditory verbal therapy was the method of choice; the implants' smooth segue into verbal language and speech production was probably based on the preimplant phonological links provided by cued speech (see Berlin et al., 1998).

Patient 3

Presenting a behavioral audiogram much like Patient 2, this 28-year-old woman claimed to be unable to hear after being beaten by her common-law husband. She was examined by a team for her husband's attorney and declared to be a malingerer because she acted so deaf and had normal emissions (Figure 8–5). Her absent middle ear muscle reflexes, which were essentially a prime warning for auditory dys-synchrony, were ignored. An ABR done with only one polarity was also understandably misinterpreted as normal at one high intensity by a neurology consultant because of a five-wave complex that appeared normal.

However, when the ABR was repeated with one positive and one negative polarity click, the waves interpreted to be normal ABR were revealed to be actually cochlear microphonics, since they inverted in polarity when the polarity of the stimulus was inverted. Normal emissions with absent middle ear muscle reflexes will almost always lead to a diagnosis of auditory neuropathy/auditory dys-synchrony.

The misdiagnosis of malingering has been removed from her record and she is being considered for a cochlear implant, although at present the mechanism by which a head injury could cause this constellation of problems remains unclear. If it were truly a central brainstem problem, she would retain a wave I in the proper polarity and only the rest of her ABR would be compromised.

This case shows that neither the ABR nor otoacoustic emissions are in and of themselves complete hearing tests but must be used together to better understand the physiology behind the audiogram. The case further highlights the value of tympanometry, followed by reflexes and emissions, for primary intake triage.

Patient 4

After local anesthesia for a dental procedure, this patient claimed to be totally deaf. Her voluntary audiometry for both speech and pure tones, done elsewhere, suggested total deafness. However, her normal emissions made it likely that more tests were necessary and she was referred to us to rule out auditory neuropathy. When we tested her with the Triage Trio, she showed normal middle ear muscle reflexes. The three tests used for triage showed that OHCs were functioning, but auditory neuropathy/dys-synchrony was not likely because the middle ear muscle reflexes were intact. Her ABR is shown in Figure 8–6 and reveals that she has normal synchrony, a normal latency intensity function, and normal cochlear function.

Since she also showed a positive delayed auditory feedback phenomenon (hesitating and prolonging words and syllables when she heard her own utterances delayed by 200 msec), we felt there was good reason to believe this was more likely to be a psychiatric case rather than an audiologic case.

DISCUSSION

Because there are at least these five events in the cochlea, and many more yet to be outlined or categorized, we know there are at least 5 ! as this ! indicates 5 factorial [5 factorial or $5 \times 4 \times 3 \times 2 \times 1$ or 120 different orders] in which cochlear events can malfunction. Some of these events (i.e., absent endocochlear potential in the presence of many other normal response) are thought to be impossible; however, since the order in which events occur may be diagnostic (e.g., the emissions and the cochlear microphonic might be present at first, but then the emissions might disappear but the cochlear microphonic would remain, or the emissions disappear and soon thereafter so do the cochlear microphonics, etc.) so the number of possible combinations is considerably less than 120.

Management should fit the physiology led by the Triage Trio more than the audiogram. The Triage Trio—tympanometry, reflexes, and emissions (TREO)—set the stage for subsequent tests and diagnostic procedures as well as interpretations. The final diagnosis and management should be consistent with these findings until we have better data to interpret the physiology behind any given audiogram and any given test result.

Immediately after birth it is possible to perform tympanometry (at high frequencies), middle ear muscle reflexes, and otoacoustic emissions. If tympanometry is dubious, but emissions are present, it is clear that the outer hair cells, middle ear, and EP are functioning. At this point a screening ABR with one positive and one negative polarity click (or even one with alternating polarity clicks for purposes of screening alone) would differentiate an ordinary cochlear loss from auditory dys-synchrony/neuropathy. The timing here is important.

A firm diagnosis cannot be made from screening data alone. Any failure of any parts of the screening test, however, should lead to a series of tests to assure a proper auditory diagnosis on or before the child's third month of life. In this way intervention, if it is needed, can minimize language delay (Yoshinaga-Itano, Sedey, Coulter, & Mehl, 1998). Waiting 3 months for another test is too long, in our opinion, due to the necessary delays in intervention thereafter.

REFERENCES

Berlin, C. I., Hood, L. J., Hurley, A., & Wen, H. (1996). Hearing aids: Only for hearing-impaired patients with abnormal otoacoustic emissions. In C. I. Berlin (Ed.), *Hair cells and hearing aids* (pp. 99–111). San Diego, CA: Singular Publishing Group.

Berlin, C. I., Bordelon, J., St. John, P., Wilensky, D., Hurley, A., Kluka, E., & Hood, L. J. (1998). Reversing click polarity may uncover auditory neuropathy in infants. *Ear and Hearing, 19*(1), 37–47.

Berlin, C. I., Hood, L. J., Goforth-Barter, L., & Bordelon, J. (1999). Clinical application of auditory efferent studies. In C. I. Berlin (Ed.), *The efferent auditory systems: Basic science and clinical applications* (pp. 1015–1124). San Diego, CA: Singular Publishing Group.

Cheatham, M. A., & Dallos, P. (1984). Summating potential (SP) tuning curves. *Hearing Research, 16*(2), 189–200.

Cornett, R. O., & Daisy, M. E. (1992). *The cued speech resource book for parents of deaf children* (1st ed., pp. xi, 820). Raleigh, NC: National Cued Speech Association.

Durrant, J. D., Wang, J., Ding, D. L., & Salvi, R. J. (1998). Are inner or outer hair cells the source of summating potentials recorded from the round window? *Journal of the Acoustical Society of America, 104*(1), 370–377.

Eggermont, J. J., & Odenthal, D. W. (1974). Action potentials and summating potentials in the normal human cochlea. *Acta Otolaryngology Supplement, 316*, 39–61.

Eilers, R. E., & Berlin, C. I. (1995). Advances in early detection of hearing loss in infants. *Current Problems in Pediatrics, 25*(2), 60–66.

Kemp, D. T. (1978). Stimulated acoustic emissions from within the human auditory system. *Journal of the Acoustical Society of America, 64*(5), 1386–1391.

Kemp, D. T. (1998). Echos of the traveling wave: Cochlear traveling wave simulation software and real time OAE viewer. In C. I. Berlin (Ed.), *Otoacoustic emissions: Basic science and clinical applications* (CD-ROM). San Diego, CA: Singular Publishing Group.

Konishi, T., Butler, R. A., & Fernandez, C. (1961). Effect of anoxia on cochlear potentials. *Journal of the Acoustical Society of America, 33*(3), 354.

Shera, C. A., & Guinan, J. J., Jr. (1999). Evoked otoacoustic emissions arise by two fundamentally different mechanisms: a taxonomy for mammalian OAEs. *Journal of the Acoustical Society of America, 105*(2, pt. 1), 782–798.

Spoendlin, H. (1985). Anatomy of cochlear innervation. *American Journal of Otolaryngology, 6*(6), 453–467.

Wever, E. G. (1959). The cochlear potentials and their relation to hearing. *Trans American Otolaryngology Society, 47*, 13–27.

Withnell, R. H. (2001). Brief report: The cochlear microphonic as an indication of outer hair cell function. *Ear & Hearing, 22*(1), 75–77.

Yoshinaga-Itano, C., Sedey, A. L., Coulter, D. K., & Mehl, A. L. (1998). Language of early- and later-identified children with hearing loss. *Pediatrics, 102*(5), 1161–1171.

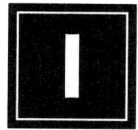

Index